FUNCTIONAL
TRAINING
FOR THE
MIND

FUNCTIONAL
TRAINING
FOR THE
MIND

How Physical Fitness Can Improve Your Focus, Mental Clarity, and Concentration

JEREMY BHANDARI

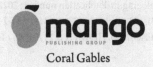

mango
PUBLISHING GROUP

Coral Gables

Published by Mango Publishing, a division of Mango Publishing Group, Inc.

Cover Design: Megan Werner
Cover illustration: AdobeStock/bloomicon
Layout & Design: Stan Info Solutions

For permission requests, please contact the publisher at:
Mango Publishing Group
2850 S Douglas Road, 4th Floor
Coral Gables, FL 33134 USA
info@mango.bz

For special orders, quantity sales, course adoptions and corporate sales, please email the publisher at sales@mango.bz. For trade and wholesale sales, please contact Ingram Publisher Services at customer.service@ingramcontent.com or +1.800.509.4887.

Functional Training for the Mind: How Physical Fitness Can Improve Your Focus, Mental Clarity, and Concentration

Library of Congress Cataloging-in-Publication number: 2022946592
ISBN: (print) 978-1-68481-133-5, (ebook) 978-1-68481-134-2
BISAC category code: HEA007050, HEALTH & FITNESS / Exercise / Strength Training

Printed in the United States of America

CONTENTS

CONTENTS

INTRODUCTION

One of the more satisfying feelings in the world earnestly emerges within each of our bodies whenever we personally accomplish something that we had specifically set out for. Whether it's a skyscraping objective like becoming an esteemed expert in an area that is widely considered difficult, or something as simple as tying our shoes, the sensation that stems from completing an intention is always deeply appreciated. So much so that, in recent years, it had me constantly pondering the following question:

How does one consistently attain whatever it is that they aim to achieve?

My initial purpose in thinking through this uncluttered, yet astonishingly complex, inquiry was not to acquire a direct answer. Don't get me wrong—solving this puzzling question would be nothing short of tremendous—but my opening intent was to candidly gain a stronger understanding of what I am asking.

To do this, I have taken action. Action in mental thought, and action as it relates to physical energy usage. Introspectively, I have spent an absurd amount of stamina analyzing the previously referenced feat of tying a pair of shoes. To eloquently explain my analysis, let's take my brand new, crisp, white Nike Air Force Ones and use them as the centerpiece of the investigation. By the time this literary piece is published, due to the number of hours that I'll end up operating in the kicks between now and then, they probably won't be as snow-colored as preferred, but that's beside the point. When putting them on, the aim, with each shoe, is to create a sturdy knot that will allow me to move with ease, which, in turn, ensures that I will not have to worry about potentially falling over due to a poorly generated loop.

With the objective understood, it is now time to take my energy and put it into action. As someone in their twenties, I can confidently say that, due to countless reps, I don't have to give too much thought to this particular deed. Without employing a ton of cerebral energy, I pick up the laces, thread one lace over its opposing counterpart, and tightly pull. Once the connection is formed in the middle of the shoe, I generate a loop with one of the laces. Holding this in place, I take my vacant hand and wrap the non-looped lace around the looped one. From here, I pull the shoelace through the concocted hole, and voila, my shoe is now tied. I repeat this act with the other tennis shoe, and now I have officially completed the task at hand.

From an unvarnished perspective, how was my ambition realized in this three-dimensional space? The answer is quite elementary: First off, I had the resources necessary for success: two pure feet, functioning fingers, and the uncontaminated shoes themselves. Additionally, although I did not enter this sphere knowing how to properly lace up a pair of kicks, I have put time and energy toward the act on innumerable occasions. This has allowed me to learn what is effective, and what's not, which has ultimately led to me mastering the procedure. The countless hours of energy spent on tying my shoes throughout my lifetime has also armed me with an unwavering belief in my ability to achieve success in the act.

From here, I can assuredly say that a ratified recipe for achieving one's aims is the following:

1. Own the appropriate resources.
2. Have a clear understanding of the ideal outcome.
3. Take consistent action to further improve your success rate when performing the act.
4. Carry an unshakeable belief in your ability to flourish in the feat.

Keep in mind, for objectives to fully materialize, you must possess an unimpeded "want" to see the specific desire come to fruition. The intensity with which you crave for something to corporealize actively influences when the intention will be revealed.

All this is great. So, since we feel marvelous when we steadily complete our missions, how do we take the shoe example, a proven victory, and duplicate this creation in all areas of our life, spanning from our ability to productively oversee our physical and mental health, to our personal power when it comes to actualizing prosperity, all the way over to the strength of our relationships with family and friends? In other words, since we've already proved that we can effectively succeed in producing our desired result, is it possible to clone this exercise and use the same strategy for whenever we would like to recognize any other particular outcome?

If the answer is yes, then how do we brand this formula and habitually utilize it throughout our daily lives without having to put too much thought into it? On any given day, we partake in countless actions where a positive or negative result is possible, making it incredibly difficult to stop and break down each scenario.

With that said, is there something that we can do during our waking hours that will instinctively stamp the success code into our consciousness to further assist us in attaining whatever it is that we long for? Yes, and that "something" is physical exercise.

While this may come as a shock to some, it has been scientifically proven that consistently exercising in any fashion is a wildly effective way to develop a strong framework for achieving desired results. This book will defend that claim and, because of its positive and educational messaging, will simultaneously uplift your mind and spirit. As someone who aspires to improve each day, I believe it is especially important to only consume content that will aid you in your personal growth. So that's what I've created for you with this product.

Before beginning, I would like to make something clear. The purpose of *Functional Training for the Mind* is not to convince you to work out more than you already do. Its sole objective is to outline how routinely exercising will inherently aid you in your pursuit of success across all areas of your life.

Each chapter will focus on a different theme that plays a role in individual achievement. Within each section, I will discuss the titled concept in depth, touching on the fitness aspect first, and then always bringing it back to our mission—which, again, is to clearly lay out how a consistent workout plan will strongly serve you when in pursuit of producing positive outcomes in all areas of your human experience. At the end of each topic, I will summarily state how the subject at hand ties into (no pun intended) the shoe example, as well as the recipe for accomplishing a goal. Think of this part of the product as a chorus in a song, utilized for repetitive purposes, to concretely ingrain the concept in your mind.

By way of design, I have done my best to speak in straightforward terms so that the information is easily absorbed. In my opinion, life is a lot simpler than our society makes it out to be, so it's important to lay out ideas in a clear, and concise, manner. To help you visualize my target as the author, let's metaphorically think of this existence as a ballpark in the midst of a summer baseball game. You, as an active being in this space, are sitting somewhere in the jam-packed crowd. Simultaneously, there are competitors battling it out on the diamond. Your fellow fans are either cheering, bantering, eating, drinking, or calmly observing, and the stadium vendors are doing their best to get your money. In the blue, cloud-filled, sky, birds are flying around, and the sun is shining bright. A lot is happening all at once. Think of this book as the sun in this scene, a beam of light that provides powerful energy amidst a sophisticated sphere.

As always, I appreciate you for the support. Let's win.

Chapter 1

LONGEVITY

For all we know, in order for an individual to manifest palpable results in this amazingly elaborate universe, the being must be filled with active energy and a lively spirit. When I say "active energy," I am referring to one's ability to physically move their muscles in accordance with all mental flares that spark within the brain whenever one consciously puts forth an effort to create corporal motion. The level at which someone feels most "alive" of course depends on the state of one's physical and mental health, but for the purpose of this book, let's proceed by assuming your body feels solid, and you are in a strong enough state of mind that you are able to assimilate these words.

To not be conscious and viable is to be lifeless, which would mean that one is unable to produce outcomes in the physical realm. The inaugural chapter in this book is titled "Longevity" because the more time we have on Earth, the more opportunities we will have to create, thus making our visceral stamina incredibly important. The sole purpose of this section is to set the foundation for the subsequent pieces, which will contain philosophical thinking mixed with science around fitness.

Excluding any external factors beyond one's control that could alter their physical and mental health, numerous studies have been published by credible sources where a correlation between exercise and longevity is profoundly present. In 2019, Harvard Health Publishing, the media and publishing division of the Medical School of Harvard University, issued an article where the author examined the relationship between fitness and mortality. In the piece, a study a study published in *The Journal of the American Medical Association* (JAMA) is referenced in which a group of academics evaluated 122,007 participants (ages ranging from eighteen to eighty, with the average age being fifty-three) on their levels of cardiorespiratory fitness (CRF). CRF, according to the American Heart Association journal *Stroke*, "refers to the capacity of the circulatory and respiratory systems to supply oxygen to skeletal muscle mitochondria for energy production needed during physical exercise." In essence, it determines how effectively someone's heart and lungs are pumping blood and oxygen throughout their being. The more in-shape someone is, the higher their level of CRF is. A measurement of something like CRF is necessary because it's tangible and provides objective value. It is a significantly stronger source of evidence than, say, a group of individuals being asked about their exercise habits. The latter is, of course, unreliable.

For this particular study, the participants were examined using the most common procedure to analyze CRF, which is exercise treadmill testing (ETT). Analyzing physical health data collected by way of a treadmill test is remarkably effective because, when one is actively moving on a treadmill, they are strengthening their cardiovascular system and intensely working the lower body muscles like the quads, thighs, hamstrings, calves, and glutes. Though not as intensely involved, abs, arms, back, shoulders, and pectoral muscles are also at work, making it relatively close to a full-body workout. To determine the difficulty level of the exercise for each individual, the participants answered a series of questions and an exercise physiologist decided on the best practice.

The testing took place from January 1, 1991, to December 31, 2014, and to properly track the analysis, each member of the group was followed up with every eight years or so during the time period. The data was reviewed in 2018, and the researchers found that a higher CRF equaled a higher survival rate. Not only did the study further prove that being in shape is linked with living longer, but it also showed that high aerobic fitness was directly proportionate with the greatest survival rate. This means that, if you choose to regularly run on a treadmill, or consistently perform any type of exercise where you are healthily increasing your heart rate, you are scientifically putting yourself in the best position possible for survival. If you habitually exercise and push yourself to the limit in those workouts, you are indisputably giving yourself the best chance for competent continuation in the cosmos, and that's marvelous.

Beyond the energy enhancement, a plethora of studies have
been published over the years that all determined that regularly
exercising significantly lowers the risk of getting diagnosed with
chronic ailments like heart disease, type 2 diabetes, arthritis,
asthma, cancer, and dementia. To justify this declaration,
academics at the Westmead Institute for Medical Research
gathered up 1,584 Australian adults, all aged over forty-nine, and
asked each participant about their weekly metabolic equivalent
minutes (METs). For accuracy purposes, none of the adults in
the study had cancer or coronary artery disease, and had never
previously suffered from a stroke.

By the way, a MET, by definition, is a unit of energy expenditure
and, like ETT, is practical to use when studying exercise habits.
One MET is roughly 3.5 milliliters of oxygen consumed per
kilogram of body weight per minute. So, if someone weighs
150 pounds (about 68 kg), then, while at rest, they would be
consuming around 238 (68 x 3.5) milliliters of oxygen per
minute. For someone around that same weight, here are a few
physical activities to help you further understand exercise in
correlation to METs.

- Washing dishes: 2.1 METs
- Briskly walking at 3 miles per hour: 3.2 METs
- Hiking at a standard rate: 6 METs
- Swimming at an average speed of 2 miles per
  hour: 8.9 METs
- Weight training (heavy weights): 10.9 METs

- Running at 8 miles per hour: 12.9 METs

This data was pulled from a publication off of Wiley.com titled "Metabolic Equivalents (METS) in Exercise Testing, Exercise Prescription, and Evaluation of Functional Capacity."

While on the subject, the World Health Organization (WHO) recommends that, at minimum, people should aim for six hundred MET minutes/week, but deeper analysis like the aforementioned study recommends getting closer to three to four thousand MET minutes/week for optimal health.

Anyways, the research team tracked the group over a ten-year period and concluded that those who exercised the most (five thousand or more MET minutes per week) were two times as likely to be free from both chronic disease and mental deterioration in comparison to those with a low weekly MET count. One of the academics who took part in analyzing the data, Bamini Gopinath, lead researcher and associate professor at the University of Sydney, expressed how the study illustrated that "high levels of physical activity increase the likelihood of surviving an extra ten years free from chronic diseases, mental impairment, and disability." In conclusion, routinely engaging in spirited physical training can provide you with an additional decade of supreme well-being.

Aside from combating extreme diseases, exercising has also consistently been proven to give individuals the upper hand

when facing less-severe bugs like the cold. In a study published
in the *British Journal of Sports Medicine*, a crew of researchers
monitored upper respiratory tract infection (URTI) symptoms
amongst a group of 1,002 adults (ages eighteen to eighty-five
years, 60 percent female, 40 percent male) for twelve weeks to
examine if physical activity played any sort of role in keeping
people free of a cough, sore throat, common cold, headache,
runny nose, or any other URTI symptom.

For each day of the experiment, the participants were required to
report on any sensed URTI symptom, and were also asked to rate
their aerobic activity habits, using a ten-point scale. In order for
an individual to appropriately announce a number on the higher
end of the scoring system, their referenced action had to qualify
as a legitimate "aerobic activity," which, per the study, meant that
the individual needed to exercise for at least twenty minutes and
the session had to be hard enough that the being would at least
break a sweat.

The statistics from the study showed that those who registered
five days or more per week of authentic aerobic activity were 43
percent less likely to experience a day with URTI symptoms than
those who reported that they exercised just one day a week or less.
In summary, physical exercise snips the possibility of coming
down with a cold by nearly 50 percent.

So far, I have emphatically explained how consistently working out helps reduce the risk of chronic ailments and other medical issues, while also proving that a nice sweat on a regular basis will enhance your day-to-day stamina levels and have a significant effect on your spirit as a whole. Now it's time to briefly touch on how exercising aids muscle growth and heart health, helps us maintain a solid weight, and why this is all meaningful for personal success.

The scientific explanation on how exercising strengthens muscle is rather intricate, but I like Young Sub Kwon and Len Kravitz's summary in their article "How Do Muscles Grow?" published on the University of Mexico's official website: "Muscle growth occurs whenever the rate of muscle protein synthesis is greater than the rate of muscle protein breakdown."

So why is it important to build muscle by way of exercising? Well, for one, whether it be lifting weights at the gym, running on a track, briskly walking around the neighborhood, going for a bike ride through town, or doing some squats in your living room, any recognized form of physical activity will help increase bone density. This is vital because, if you have weak bones, you are not only putting yourself at risk for osteoporosis, but you're also increasing the odds that you'll suffer from a bone break. Beyond the physical ramifications, a broken bone means time and energy taken away from your everyday life, which is detrimental in the pursuit of success across any endeavor. Humans naturally lose muscle as they get older, and it is believed that by age thirty, we start to lose up to 3 to 5 percent of muscle per every succeeding decade, making a focus on steady exercise that much more crucial.

Now, a few words on the importance of having a healthy heart. Heart disease is, by far, the leading cause of death in this world. In the United States alone, the Centers for Disease Control and Prevention (CDC) claims that about 659,000 people die from heart disease each year. It's estimated that someone dies every thirty-six seconds in this nation from heart disease. These facts alone should trigger something inside your soul to do everything in your power to keep your heart as strong as humanly possible.

Fortunately, one of the most effective sets of actions we can take to keep our hearts in peak form is, of course, consistently exercising. Whenever you run, swim, jump rope, or perform any other aerobic exercise, you are naturally boosting your circulation. An enhancement in circulation improves blood flow, which allows for the heart to productively pump blood to distribute oxygen and nutrients to the other areas of the body.

When you lift free weights at the gym, use any of the weight machines, do pull-ups, or simply drop down on all fours to perform a set of push-ups, you are effectively increasing your HDL (high-density lipoprotein) cholesterol and lowering your LDL (low-density lipoprotein) cholesterol. For those who are unfamiliar, HDL is the "good" kind of cholesterol, and LDL is the "bad" kind. If you build up enough "bad" cholesterol in your blood, you are putting yourself at risk for cardiovascular disease.

From an overarching perspective, the strength of your heart not only influences the effectiveness of your breathing, but also has a direct impact on your energy levels. Low energy levels lead to fatigue. Being fatigued can snowball into a headache, dizziness, inability to focus, moodiness, and a surplus of other physical, mental, and emotional issues. Suffering from any of these symptoms will immediately put you at a severe disadvantage when on the pursuit of accomplishing your desires.

To sum up the above discussion, exercising efficiently enhances your energy levels, improves blood flow, is wildly effective for developing bone and muscle strength, lowers LDL cholesterol, strengthens your heart, and prevents you from getting sick by any stretch of the definition.

Finally, the obvious statement: Working out helps you maintain a good body weight. The more consistent you are with your workouts, the easier it is to preserve, protect, and prolong your physical powers. Speaking figuratively, sustaining a fit body is like keeping up a fresh, radiant yard of green grass. In order to prolong the grass's green glow, one must constantly care for it. If one chooses to neglect the patch for an extended amount of time, the sparkle and overall spirit will be sorrowfully drained out of the yard, and the gloomy results will be in plain sight. Therefore, all stamina spent toward physical movement directly benefits the body by keeping it fit as a fiddle, just as any energy put toward nurturing a grassy meadow helps the space remain healthy and strong.

When discussing obesity, a common measurement that often gets cited is body-mass index (BMI), which, by its dictionary definition, is a weight-to-height ratio, calculated by dividing one's weight in kilograms by the square of one's height in meters. While it's obviously not an impeccable computation to determine body fat, especially for highly active beings with dense muscle and bones, measuring BMI helps detect whether someone is at a healthy weight or not.

A healthy BMI range, according to the World Health Organization, is anywhere between 18.5 and 24.9. Those who fall between 25 and 29.9 are considered "overweight," and anyone above 30 would be marked "obese."

For some statistical context on both historical and present data around body fat, here is a mind-boggling fact. In the early 1960s, less than 14 percent of people in the United States walked around with a BMI over 30. Today, that number is right around 40 percent. As an avid baseball fan, I take great joy in hopping on YouTube to watch video footage of early 1960s ballgames where stars like Willie Mays and Mickey Mantle excelled in

the major leagues. Whenever I watch either of them round the
bases after a towering home run, I always hone in on the crowd's
energy—mainly to see just how influential these legends were in
their heyday, but I also like to get a reminder of what watching a
sporting event was like before cell phones. My general takeaway is
always the same: Those fans, in comparison to today's followers,
seemed more present and appeared to genuinely appreciate what
they were witnessing. That might be accurate, but what's an actual
fact is that those enthusiasts who were passionately supporting
Mays and Mantle were around three times less likely to be obese
than present-day admirers, which certainly plays a role in their
level of engagement and overall excitement.

The litany of consequences that come with carrying excess body
fat have been profusely documented over the years, and, sadly, as
time goes on, that list of negative implications continues to grow.
In short, an overweight individual puts themselves at a severe
health risk for the following: Type 2 diabetes, high blood pressure,
heart disease, hardened arteries, sleep apnea, gout, gallstones,
osteoarthritis, liver disease, kidney disease, some forms of cancer,
and many more extreme conditions. In the United States alone, it
is estimated that obesity kills around 300,000 people per year.

While that number is surely alarming, it should be made clear
that, for many of us, managing one's weight is totally up to the
being in the body. In fact, according to the National Institutes
of Health, the second leading cause of preventable death in the

United States is obesity and overweight together, trailing only tobacco use for the crown in that category.

Since our job as alert, conscious souls is to maintain a healthy weight, what is the most effective action to take during our waking hours to ensure we are in the best position for success in this department? Exercise.

For the longest time, the initial thought following an obesity or overweight diagnosis was to lock in on the idea of shedding the superfluous pounds by mapping out a diet to follow for a set amount of days. However, in a 2021 review article published in *iScience*, present-day researchers firmly believe that, to adequately reach a healthy weight, individuals should primarily focus on increasing their overall physical activity levels by bettering their fitness routine. The authors in the publication encourage readers to put an emphasis on exercising instead of a drastic dietary change because the latter has proven to be ineffective. If the spotlight is on nutrition, overweight individuals will typically launch an extreme diet plan, which, at first, appears to be practical. For most, the changes in food choice and overall caloric intake will for sure lead to weight loss. However, as time prolongs, the massive alterations that came with the new diet can shock the system and lead to negative effects like depression or fatigue. This creates a hamster wheel, or what's typically called a "yo-yo diet," where the individual begins the diet and sees positive results, but has created such intense boundaries in regard to their food choices that they almost always spiral back to their old ways and, not just gain the weight back, but in many situations, put on even more pounds than they had before because of the emotional complications spawned by the severe regimen. Beyond adding the weight back on and potentially creating feelings of despair and weariness, partaking in a yo-yo diet has also been associated with major health problems like muscle loss, fatty liver disease, and diabetes.

In the review, the research team fixated on their claim, pulled from recent mortality risk reduction data, and concluded that the risk reduction connected with calculated weight loss was frequently lower than that associated with an increase in physical activity levels. This, of course, should come as no surprise because, unlike the physical and emotional effects that could stem from an intense diet, exercising naturally strengthens the body and generates powerful feelings of positivity.

Now, this is not to say that nutrition should be ignored or neglected, by any means, when on the path to living a healthy, happy, successful life. Nutrition is incredibly important—so much so that I meticulously thought about turning this product into a fitness and nutrition book, but both categories are so dense that I would be doing a disservice to each if I divided the information up. Also, trying to productively provide dietary advice is difficult because meal plans vary drastically depending on lifestyle. Two people could be the same age, and have identical physical measurements, but if one is in the NFL, and the other primarily works a desk job, they are completely incomparable from a nutrition standpoint because of the contrasting energy habits that come from the two occupations.

However, since it's always beneficial to be reminded of the positive foods in life, I will occasionally bring up nutrition if it's universally recognized as a strong option in relation to the topic we are discussing. For example, when it comes to healthy bone growth, in conjunction with consistently exercising, dairy products such as yogurt, milk, and cheese are great options because of their high calcium content. In past publications, the US Department of Agriculture has referenced both a cup of fat-free milk and a cup of plain nonfat Greek yogurt as two strong sources of calcium. If you are like me, and aren't a fan of consuming plain yogurt by itself, I highly recommend including it as a staple in a morning smoothie.

In addition to dairy products, other calcium-rich options include plant-based foods like broccoli, spinach, cabbage, okra, black beans, edamame, pinto beans, kidney beans, tofu, chia seeds, flaxseed, pumpkin seeds, sesame seeds, and nuts. All the catalogued bean choices, along with nuts like almonds, peanuts, walnuts, and pecans, are great selections because they all contain high levels of magnesium and phosphorus, which are both imperative to bone health.

To ensure productive bone growth, aside from a focus on calcium consumption, nutritionists also recommend concentrating on your daily vitamin D intake. However, very few foods are naturally packed with vitamin D, making it incredibly difficult to reach the recommended daily amount of six hundred IU (international units). In fact, vitamin D is so scarce in food that around 42 percent of the US population is considered vitamin D-deficient. In my humble opinion, this feels like an issue that should be further discussed on a national level.

Among the limited amount of food that is rich in vitamin D, cod liver oil, salmon, swordfish, and tuna are going to be your best options. Eating egg yolks and beef liver will also help you work toward your daily intake aim, but, even if you consumed one of the listed items in each of your meals, you would still most likely fall short of your goal, which is why a vitamin D supplement is highly recommended. Personally, I like the supplements created by Thorne, a practitioner-trusted brand. One pill contains a thousand IU, making it remarkably easy to surpass the advised daily intake.

Spotlighting heart health, fruits and vegetables, whole grains, low-fat dairy products, skinless poultry, fish, nuts and beans, and non-tropical vegetable oils have all been proven to be viable options.

In regard to muscle growth, the universal prescription is to eat healthy foods that are rich in protein. Carbohydrates and fats also play a notable role in this space, but protein consumption is unquestionably considered the main component when it comes to developing strong muscles. A few hearty options have already been referenced, but foods like eggs, salmon, chicken breast, lean beef, Greek yogurt, tuna, shrimp, soybeans, chickpeas, and tofu, to name a few, are all tremendous choices for high protein consumption.

All of the cited nourishment options obviously aid with longevity as a whole, so a primary focus on these nutritious selections will certainly put you in an outstanding position for long-term success. Aside from that, the only other necessary piece of advice would be to do your very best to only consume products, either independently or mixed with other exquisite eats, that contain just one ingredient. For example, when you bite into a juicy, red apple, you are distinctly chewing on the contents of a round fruit that originated from a tree of the rose family. On the flip side, if you choose to eat a prepackaged cinnamon roll, though it might be more delectable than a piece of fruit, just know that you are loading up your body with the following ingredients: Enriched Flour Bleached, Sugar, Palm and Soybean Oil, Dextrose, Wheat Starch, Modified Whey, Corn Syrup Solids, Cinnamon, Monoglycerides, Xanthan Gum, Potassium Sorbate, Polylobate 60, Corn Starch, Natural and Artificial Flavor, and Annatto Extract. Now, I'm certainly no nutritionist, but even without a formal education in the field, I can confidently say that a lion's share of those ingredients do not belong in our being. Long story short, eat real food, and, if consuming a packaged nourishment option, take a few seconds out of your day to scan the product's contents before masticating.

Now that the groundwork for this book's focus has been conscientiously and passionately laid out between the paper's lines, let's tie the importance of this section in to the previously mentioned Shoe Theory to further illuminate how routinely exercising is an astonishingly powerful action to take when on the pursuit for personal prosperity. Throughout the chapter, utilizing both fixed science and extensive human trial-and-error, it's clear that working out will undeniably put you in the best physical position to energetically engage with the world. Bodily strength is of supreme significance in this sphere because, if you do not feel good from a physical standpoint, your overall output will suffer. Let's say you bend down to tie your shoes, and, in the process, your body aches. Depending on the severity of the soreness, you still will most likely be able to accomplish the goal of fittingly lacing your shoes. However, had your body been at 100 percent when you took the action, you would have performed in a more enjoyable and effective manner.

Even though it's an elementary example, the thought process is directly applicable with any aim that you set. If you're an athlete in competition who aspires to put up particular individual statistics or play a significant role in helping your team win a championship, you will be at a substantial disadvantage to your counterparts if you aren't fully healthy. Beyond sports, if you're someone who is starting a business with the hopes of launching a compelling product or service, you'll be required to exhaust considerable energy in the course of spending countless hours on your concept. Heck, even if the target is to develop a stronger relationship with a coworker, partner, friend, or family member, your physical health plays a major role in how you develop the connection. You don't feel good if you don't feel good, which sounds like an incredibly witless and primitive statement, but it's the flat-out truth.

Just think back on past moments in your life in which you achieved positive results that you're proud of. Close your eyes and envision the exact moment of gratification in any of those instances. I would have to imagine that in most, if not all scenarios, you felt alive and fresh. Again, all we are attempting to do in this experience is consistently manifest whatever it is that we desire in the present moment. After analyzing our past favorable realizations, it is clear that physical health plays an essential part in the result. Knowing this, as we saunter on through the various stages of life, a rational intention throughout this amusing adventure would be to take the appropriate actions that put us in the best position to consistently feel physically fit.

In reference to the previously hatched recipe for reward in this realm, physical health contributes to both rules one and three. You can't "own the appropriate resources" if you aren't effectively existing in the flesh, and the degree to which you improve when you take consistent action on your aim is directly correlated with how you feel when pursuing the undertaking. If you've ever taken the time to do some research on the longest-living people, then you've surely stumbled across the Ikarians of Greece or the Okinawans of Japan. In both societies, whether it's an everyday focus on gardening, walking, or any other activity that requires bodily motion, the plurality of people operating in these civilizations make a purposeful effort to stay physically active on a daily basis, which allows us to confidently conclude that deliberately moving around throughout our day will surely strengthen our ability to continuously create.

As a whole, if a person wishes to persistently pursue ambitious aims over a protracted period of time, they must ensure that their physical body is as close to 100 percent health as humanly possible. Regularly exercising will not only actively aid in boosting your bodily being, but, as we will soon find, it's also an astonishingly effective activity to enhance your sagacity.

Chapter 2

SAGACITY

The word *sagacity* is defined as "acuteness of mental discernment and soundness of judgement." For this special section, I will be covering mental wisdom as a whole, and explain how fitness links with brain power.

An individual's ability to amass and administer intelligence and artistry is unequivocally influenced by, not only where their energy is spent during their waking hours, but also what their level of focus is on the task or act that they wish to improve on. I will be covering "focus" as its own entity in a later chapter, so for now, the objective is to touch on the relationship between working out and mental intelligence, while also outlining the importance of acumen when it comes to achieving our ambitions.

If someone is considered "intelligent" or "skilled" in a specific field, it really means that they have a strong understanding of the ins and outs of that discipline, which allows them to efficiently put energy toward the craft and, in return, receive positive results. To reach "master" status in an area, one must exhaust an immeasurable amount of energy in the desired discipline. This means repeating acts over and over until they are perfected.

So let's start with the concept of repetition. A typical workout plan consists of various exercises in which each drill is independently broken down into a handful of sets. It is wildly common, especially when weight training, to perform three sets of whatever activity you are presently partaking in. For example, if you were doing bicep curls, then you could do three sets of ten reps to effectively enhance your arms' flexibility and strength. The number of reps for any exercise is exclusively dependent on the objective. Ten is practically always a good number for perceptible results, but, if you're looking to specifically improve endurance, then twelve to fifteen reps of a light load would be more effective. If strength is a main point of focus, then doing three to five reps of heavy weight would be suitable. No matter what, through fitness, your being is regularly repeating the same actions over and over again, which, surprisingly, does wonders for your mind.

Our brain, on average, has eighty-six billion neurons. These neurons effectively communicate with each other via electrical signals known as "action potentials" and chemical neurotransmitters. The three preeminent parts within each neuron that allow for cogent communication are the dendrites, the cell body, and the axon. The dendrite receives the electrical message, the cell body deciphers the message, and the axon, a cytoplasmic protrusion from the cell body, essentially serves as a rope and carries the signal to the adjacent neuron.

There is a lipid-rich material that armors the axon, called myelin, which serves as insulation. A common way to comprehend this information is likening the process to an iPhone charger. Metaphorically, the neuron serves as the power plug, the axon as the operating wire, and the myelin as the rubber insulation. Phone chargers are at their best when the rubber perfectly shields the wire, and the brain is no different. When the axon is effectively sheltered, the signal travels at a strong rate from one neuron to the next. The quicker the neurons communicate with each other, the easier it is to execute on the act.

Academics in this area believe that repeating an action leads to an increase in myelin around the structure, which naturally translates to improved brain function. So, when someone says "practice makes perfect," they are essentially stating that the more you do something, the better you become, because repetition ensures that your neurons are communicating as efficiently as possible. This should come as no surprise, but it's nice to put science to the idea of improving by performing an act over and over.

Duplicating actions by way of a fitness routine is highly effective because, not only are you boosting your physical health with each rep, but at the same time, you're scientifically enhancing the rate at which you comprehend information. When you work out, you naturally improve the effectiveness of your neuromuscular system. Before you move a particular muscle, your brain must first drop a signal down to the nerve in that specified bundle of fibrous tissue. Then, the desired action can occur in which the movement takes place. The more reps we get in the gym, the better our brain gets at signaling our bodies to perform the act. Eventually, if we perform the same exercise over and over on a consistent basis, it becomes "muscle memory," which is a rudimentary phrase to use when someone has a strong brain-body connection whenever they put energy toward an explicit physical move. Think about Steph Curry rather effortlessly swishing a three-point field goal. Or the late-great Prince smoothly rocking out on stage. At the core, their neuromuscular systems, which were developed through an insane number of reps, deserve all the credit for their ability to flourish in their specialized fields.

Humans are creatures of habit, so by partaking in an exercise routine in which you are regularly performing the same drill, you are not only building up your mental aptitude, but you're also skillfully programming your mind with a pattern to follow for any future endeavor that you wish to engage in. Since exercising creates a positive feeling for both body and mind, your brain will naturally suggest repetition as a powerful solution whenever you are looking to constantly achieve a desired result.

To help clarify this concept using real data, let's briefly analyze Michael Jordan, an immortal member of the Naismith Memorial Basketball Hall of Fame, who many consider to be the greatest basketball player of all time. His list of accomplishments on the court is far too extensive to cover in this project, but, in a summary that still doesn't do justice to his prominence, Jordan led the league in scoring in ten seasons, won six championships with the Chicago Bulls, and was recognized as the Most Valuable Player in the league on five separate occasions.

Zoning in on scoring in particular, Air Jordan has the most points per game (30.1 PPG) in NBA regular season history, and he also wears the crown as the player with the most points per game in NBA Playoff history (33.4 PPG). No matter the opponent, time of year, or significance of the match, Jordan got buckets. So much so that one could confidently conclude that he had a brilliant basketball mind, and developed an otherworldly talent.

So how did he progress his aptitude for scoring? Repetitive action in his discipline and impeccable mental focus. Jordan was not only scoring more than anyone, but, in his 1,072 career regular-season battles, "Black Jesus" attempted 22.9 field goals per game, which was the highest average among any player who competed during the years in which Jordan was active. He shot the ball so much that he actually led the league in misses in seven of his fifteen seasons. This stat sounds like a negative one, but, in actuality, each time Jordan shot the orange inflated ball up toward the hoop, he was improving his basketball intelligence. With every attempt, the goal was to put the ball in the hole. After each shot, Jordan's mind was instinctively taking notes, and inherently drawing up the right recipe needed to ensure that he would be in the best position possible to reach his aim. To make a long story short, the sheer volume of shots directly enhanced his understanding of how to score with the ball at the professional level, which, in turn, generated the mighty statistics.

The enhancement in brilliance through reiterative action can also be examined in the case of Ichiro Suzuki, a legendary baseball player who competed professionally in both Japan and North America. To date, Ichiro is the only hitter in Major League Baseball (MLB) history to record at least two hundred hits in ten straight seasons. Amidst his epic streak, Ichiro set the record for most hits in a single year (262 in 2004), breaking George Sisler's previous chart-topping figure of 257, which he set all the way back in 1920. What is even crazier about Ichiro stealing Sisler's crown is the fact that no ballplayer since 1930 had even amassed 250 hits within a single season, which, for a long time, had baseball historians assuming that Sisler's feat would never be surpassed.

So how did Ichiro snap an eighty-four-year-old record that appeared impossible to grasp? Well, over the course of his first three seasons in MLB (2001–03), the star outfielder went up to the plate a total of 2,191 times, which was more than any other player in the league over that span. Following each plate appearance, Ichiro's mind, nearly identical to Jordan's in the goal-setting sense, was gathering up data and effectively calculating how he could be in the strongest position for achievement for the next time that he stepped into the batter's box. By the time 2004 rolled around, his mind and body had been put in that specific success/failure situation more than anyone else in recent years, which put him in an incredible spot to consistently hit his target.

Quite obviously, there are countless of other factors as to why Ichiro and Jordan were exceptionally successful and set records, beyond just gaining mental intelligence through consistent action: physical gifts, health, luck, timing, love for the game, freakish level of self-discipline when it came to training, competitive spirit, and self-confidence, just to name a few—but that's not the point. I referenced these two because their impressive output in their professions helps illustrate how repetition in a particular field plays a vital role in achieving greatness. Concrete data is the strongest way to defend any claim, and professional sports is one of the few careers that publicly tracks performance through statistics, which allows us to efficiently exemplify specific points. Just saying that someone "put in a lot of work" as the core reason as to how they achieved success in an area is one thing, but to have tangible numbers that track individual success rates year by year, while also drawing direct comparisons to the competition, allows us to confidently surmise that repeating acts at a high rate directly enhances someone's level of mental intelligence, which, quite evidently, is an important factor in winning.

Not everyone who reads this book has dreams of starring in the NBA or MLB, but each of us would like to succeed in whatever it is that we put energy toward. Jordan and Ichiro's respective paths prove the power of mental development when one is on the pursuit for prosperity in any area that they specifically set an intention in. Michael's goal of scoring the basketball when he shoots and Ichiro's aim of getting a hit when he steps up to the plate are no different than whatever ambitions you decide upon for yourself. From a broad point of view, they put energy toward their aim at a higher rate than their competition, which naturally improved their odds of success. More time spent on your craft leads to an enhancement in understanding in that pursuit, which directly equates to a rise in mental intelligence.

Beyond aiding your mind from a repetition perspective, a study conducted at the University of British Columbia found that habitually performing an aerobic exercise has the power to boost the size of a person's hippocampus. This conclusion was reached following a six-month experiment where eighty-six adult females underwent a physical training program, while also having their attention, memory, and learning abilities evaluated by way of the Rey Auditory Verbal Learning Test. Using a 3T MRI scan, participants had their hippocampi measured at both the beginning and the end of the evaluation. In the latter analysis, the women experienced a significant size increase with respect to the entirety of their hippocampus, which naturally played a direct role in bettering their test scores. For those unfamiliar with the complex structure, it's the area in the brain that helps humans process and retrieve memory, and it is also heavily associated with learning. Oddly enough, in past research, the capacity of a hippocampus has been connected positively with IQ, so one could infer that regularly exercising plays an active role in elevating the level of one's human intelligence. Furthermore, while the majority of regions in the brain do not generate new neurons after we are born, the hippocampus is a rare exception, as adult neurogenesis is essential for certain modes of learning and memory. However, as we get older, the creation of these neurons gradually decreases, which naturally affects our ability to retain and recall information. Yet, as outlined in this study, if you routinely exercise, your brain will continue to grow and develop new nervous tissue within the hippocampus, allowing you to stay mentally sharp, even if you've celebrated more birthdays than Barry Bonds hit home runs in 2001.

Along with specifically enhancing the functionality and physical size of your hippocampus, consistently working out has also been associated with both larger rostral middle frontal volumes, and bigger orbitofrontal cortex volumes. For those unaccustomed to these regions, the rostral middle frontal gyrus (RMFG) is crucial for overall executive function, including mood regulation, running memory, and self-control. The orbitofrontal cortex is essentially a link for sensory integration, which is a fancy term used to explain the happenings in our brain that allow us to comprehend, and conclusively react to, anything that we touch, see, hear, smell, or taste. Additionally, this area in the frontal lobes of the brain is also connected with how we learn, and ultimately make decisions for both emotional and benefit-related behaviors.

In the previous chapter, I briefly touched on consistent exercise being of great benefit to the heart. A habitual workout naturally bolsters the blood-pumping organ, but, beyond the physical perks, recent studies have shown that a stronger heart helps keep the brain blossoming. Amidst a spirited run, your heart will beat faster than normal, and circulation will increase, which gets oxygenated blood to your muscles quicker. In addition, a significant amount of oxygen is sent directly to your brain. Effectively oxygenating the brain is vital to stimulate both healing and overall functionality of the astonishing three-pound organ. These facts were further analyzed in a 2016 study, titled "Fitness and cognition in the elderly," which involved 877 adults, all between the ages of fifty-eight and seventy-two. Participants exercised on a treadmill, had their oxygen levels measured by VO_2 max (maximum rate of oxygen consumption measured during a cumulative workout; a high VO_2 max means strong physical fitness, and vice versa), and partook in a series of tests to judge cerebral function. At the end of the experiment, the researchers found that higher VO_2 max was directly linked with strong cognitive function, specifically memory, motor skills, and mental abilities like time management, planning, and organizing.

With a similar focus in mind, in an examination published back in 2014, a group of intellectuals investigated how engaging in Tai

Chi, a Chinese martial art practice that is commonly rehearsed for defense training, can have an impact on overall cognitive performance in adults. For their study, a troop of humans practiced Tai Chi over a fixed period of time, and, throughout the experiment, had their cognitive abilities measured by way of neuropsychological testing.

It turns out that, in near-identical results to the previous study, according to the Harvard Health Publishing blog titled "Exercise can boost your memory and thinking skills," "tai chi showed the potential to enhance cognitive function in older adults, especially in the realm of executive function, which manages cognitive processes such as planning, working memory, attention, problem solving, and verbal reasoning."

This is influential because, when training for Tai Chi, humans are simultaneously working their upper extremity bones (upper arm, forearm, and hand), their lower extremity bones (thigh bone, shin bone, and foot), and the primary muscles of their backs and abdomens. Beyond the physical enhancement, the art calls for learning new skills and patterns, forcing the being to think outside of the box. I say this because, in any full body workout, a being will work out all of those muscles and be forced to develop the proper form for whatever exercise they partake in, which allows us to conclude with conviction that exercising as a whole will mirror the positive cognitive function effects found in adults who practiced Tai Chi.

In summary, repeating an act will improve the speed of our neurons, which enhances intelligence and overall understanding in whatever it is that we are focusing on. Because of its physical and mental benefits, effective repetition is a skill that is best developed through fitness. In just a sixty-minute workout, one could easily do a string of ten separate exercises, where repetitive sets are required for each act. The sheer amount of time spent duplicating movements in just one workout allows for the art of repetition to be developed at an incredible rate. Getting a strong grasp on how to efficiently repeat acts through fitness training will directly improve your chances of successfully echoing any activity. Aside from using repetition as a way to improve from a mental perspective, the studies referenced have shown that a consistent aerobic workout will directly boost memory and learning, while also appearing to amplify important cognitive processes.

Concisely touching on nutrition, research suggests that regularly consuming colorful vegetables may aid in slowing down cognitive decline that lamentably comes with aging. A serving a day of leafy greens like spinach, broccoli, kale, Brussels sprouts, cabbage, and lettuce, or any other vitamin K-rich food, is adequate to reap the benefits. In addition, foods that are full of beta-carotene, like carrots, sweet potatoes, butternut squash, cantaloupe, and red bell peppers, are also all great options when it comes to eating to keep your mind sharp.

With regard to improving thought retention, the most effective
nutritional option appears to be berries, or any other foods
that are high in flavonoids. This conclusion was captured in
an extensive study published in 2012 by *Annals of Neurology*,
a journal of the American Neurological Association and Child
Neurology Society. The comprehensive experiment began in
1976, when a group of Harvard researchers at Brigham and
Women's Hospital recruited 121,700 females who were all
registered nurses (RN) by profession. Starting that same year,
the participants in the test, all aged between thirty and fifty-five,
filled out health and lifestyle questionnaires to set the stage.
Since 1980, the year that our fellow humans universally mourned
over the tragic assassination of former Beatle John Lennon, the
RNs were polled every four years with respect to their frequency
of food consumption. Between 1995 and 2001, 16,010 of the
women had their memory examined at two-year intervals. Once
the data was analyzed, the intellects found that the women who
possessed slower rates of memory decline were predominately
individuals who consistently consumed the most blueberries and
strawberries. The research team also concluded that a diet with
high berry intake appeared to delay memory decline by up to two
and a half years.

For intelligent snacking purposes, an interesting study from
UCLA found positive associations between walnut consumption
and overall cognitive function. Walnuts are the only tree nut that
contain a large amount of alpha-linolenic acid (ALA), which

is a type of omega-3 fatty acid that has been linked with brain development and function. Other foods that provide substantial amounts of omega-3 fatty acids include cold-water fatty fish like salmon, mackerel, tuna, herring, and sardines, as well as plant oils, flaxseeds, and chia seeds.

Now back to the beloved Shoe Theory. As mentioned in the introduction, when we all first attempted to tie our shoes, we were collectively unsure how to best string the knots together. However, through repetition, our awareness of the concept continuously increased and eventually reached "expert" status. The understanding of how to successfully complete the action is molded into our consciousness, and, barring any major cerebral injury, will remain there for good. The time and energy it takes to reach "expert" status in any field varies drastically and depends solely on the operation, but the fabric for accelerating insight on any act is identical to tying your shoes.

This section highlighted rules two, three, and four in our recipe for success in any endeavor. In order to be in alignment with the second principle, "Have a clear understanding of the ideal outcome," our brain must be operating at a strong-enough capacity to clearly process moves, effectively retain information, and, most importantly, continuously develop intelligence in our desired area. If achieving your aim would significantly impact the specific field you're putting energy toward, then you're more than likely either competing against thousands of other individuals, or, in the rare case, attempting to do something so exclusive that it has yet to materialize because it's been undervalued or is simply too problematic for people to pursue. In plain terms, if you're up against countless other individuals who are all gunning for the same goal, then that means you're going head-to-head with a whole lot of minds. With each hour spent gaining sense in the space, a being takes a productive stride and inches closer to realization. If you do not put in the time to learn about your craft, you will get obliterated by those who steadily study. Knowing this, it becomes ever-so-vital to cultivate a high-powered mind. Fortunately, through the aforementioned scientific examinations, it is evident that regularly exercising will aid us in precisely reaching this objective.

Rule number three, "Take consistent action to further improve your success rate when performing the act" is the most marked guideline in this chapter, as the titled order could also be read as "repeat acts over and over until they are mastered." In the words of the legendary hip-hop recording artist, Lil Wayne, "repetition is the father of learning. I repeat, repetition is the father of learning. Awareness, preparation, all that comes from repetition."

Last but not least, rule number four, "Carry an unshakeable belief in your ability to flourish in the feat," played a lively role in this chunk of philosophical and scientific thought because we were able to objectively confirm that the brain, when focused on an action, instinctively works toward the desired end result and, with every occurrence, gains a progressively better understanding of the target. This, in turn, enhances belief in the strength we have to accomplish the aim. Putting in the time in your sought-after space is a necessity for intellectual growth in that arena, but now, let's take it a step further, and look into how fitness helps boost one's self-belief across all areas of life.

Chapter 3

SELF-PERCEPTION

It's really important to love yourself. Abiding self-affection helps us progress as individual people, but it's also an amazingly meaningful trait to possess as we interface with other humans. The level of self-love that one carries plays an active role in the degree to which that being can positively impact others. A strong, unwavering appreciation for oneself leads to an increase in value added to all those around.

On the flip side, if you don't have adoration and true admiration for yourself as a lively being, this adventure isn't much fun. Knowing this, it's important to do everything in our power to make sure that we develop the beneficial habits and proper thinking patterns to suitably succeed in this voyage. Life is a complex and ever-changing experience, making it impossible to remain in one concrete state of mind throughout the journey, so the fundamental aim must be to customarily take the preferred set of actions that will put us in the best position to feel exceptional in the present moment.

One of the central elements in feeling pleasant is ensuring that we predominately possess positive thoughts in our consciousness.

When we constantly think on the bright side, we begin to feel
great about, not just who we are as a being, but also what we
can sew up in this sphere. Believe it or not, every time a human
generates a thought, a chemical is discharged. When we think
positively, our brain produces serotonin, which spawns the
feeling of happiness that is sensed throughout our souls. Positive
emotions directly influence the prefrontal cortex, the cerebral
cortex covering the front part of the frontal lobe. This section of
the brain has a strong hand in influencing level of focus, mapping
complex cognitive behavior, creative thinking, and personality
expression, and also helps with modulating social behavior. The
prefrontal cortex impacts our behaviors more than any other
region in the brain, as it's where all mind-body affairs adjoin and
then get beamed to other areas of the being. Because of its high
level of influence, the prefrontal cortex controls the completion,
formation, and timing of successive actions that one takes in
pursuit of a goal. When we construct a favorable thought, there is
growth in this area of the brain through coating and cultivation of
new synapses. A resolutely activated prefrontal cortex leads to an
enhancement in effective motion and overall ardor.

Think of positive thoughts as plant seeds. As a healthy, conscious
being, you metaphorically own a garden with an abundant
amount of space to cultivate whatever it is that you desire. When
we think positively about something that we wish to experience
in reality—whether it's a personal goal coming true, working
in a dream career, or cherishing a purposeful relationship—

our prefrontal cortex naturally begins to dig up an area in our personal patch to help manifest a miraculous creation. From there, the seeds are dropped down into an allegorical dirt pit, and, through consistent efforts in producing productive thoughts, the seeds become supernatural, which allows you to instinctively make the precise choices and take the paramount actions that are needed to see your conception come to fruition. This process, in due time, like the birth of a tree, leads to palpable procreation.

Generate positive thoughts, get positive results. Think negative, get negative outcomes. This feels universally understood, but to add science to the mix, researchers from the Institute of Psychiatry, Psychology and Neuroscience (IoPPN) at King's College London compiled a research study where the primary focus of the experiment was to see if repetitive negative thinking (RNT) played a part in increasing the risk of developing Alzheimer's. Following the evaluation, the research team concluded that RNT directly impacts the brain's ability to think, reason, and form memories, which proved that consistently thinking poorly does in fact influence the risk of getting diagnosed with Alzheimer's.

Knowing the value of forward-looking thoughts, one could confidently concur that a focus on serotonin would be highly useful to an individual who is looking to improve their inner dialogue and overall internal breakdown of beliefs. An effective way to increase serotonin production is partaking in an aerobic exercise. Scientifically speaking, performing high-impact workouts, like running, swimming, stair climbing, elliptical training, biking, or rowing calls for an initiation of branched-chain amino acids. These organic compounds are ordinarily in competition with tryptophan—an amino acid used to enhance the levels of the ever-so-powerful monoamine neurotransmitter that is serotonin—to be lugged across the blood-brain barrier. When you perform any of the listed aerobic exercises, preferably for at least thirty minutes, you are naturally decreasing the amount of competitive amino acids, which, in turn, enhances tryptophan's odds of effectively crossing the blood-brain barrier. As it makes its way across this hurdle, serotonin gets sent to the brain. Something like weight lifting will also raise tryptophan, but an aerobic workout will be more impactful when it comes to generating serotonin, as your heart and lungs are put to the test more per minute in a run as opposed to a set of shoulder shrugs.

Although you can't directly get serotonin from what you eat, you can consume healthy options like salmon, poultry, eggs, dark green leafy vegetables, nuts, seeds, and oats, which are all high in tryptophan.

Staying on the topic of neurotransmitters, exercising in any fashion will also escalate the production of dopamine, which raises our feelings of pleasure and happiness. Because of its omnipotent relationship with these signaling molecules, physical training will intuitively help you think more clearly, which leads to better decision-making, which steers your soul in the right direction to take the correct action. A proper mindset, mixed with effective moves, leads to dominant results.

On top of assisting with the navigation of thoughts and actions, the dopamine release from a vigorous workout creates feelings of delight and satisfaction, which forcibly curbs the spirit from feeling anxious, stressed, or depressed.

Along with concentrating on creating, curating, and controlling all thoughts that enter our consciousness, one must also zero in on their level of self-confidence to expertly sharpen their mind. Molding a positive image in your imagination is a great start, but, if you lack internal faith in the idea's chance to fully materialize, you put yourself at a significant disadvantage.

By its formal description, self-confidence is a state of being where one possesses a strong feeling of faith in their abilities, personal qualities, and overall judgement. Since it isn't an anchored attribute, our self-confidence status must be continually supervised. Whether it's trust in ourselves to perform an action or faith in who we are as a human being, it's immensely valuable to hold a high level of self-belief in whatever we put energy toward, because what we accept to be a fact in our minds will naturally form as the truth in our reality. Our confidence levels operate as a double-edged sword. On one hand, if you carry an abundance of belief in yourself to succeed in whatever it is that you're striving for, you'll put yourself in a favorable position. Alternatively, if you enter a situation thinking that you'll fail to reach the desired target, you handicap yourself before the race has even begun. The region in our brain that primarily assists with governing our beliefs is the hippocampus, which, as we know, is positively influenced while a being is habitually exercising.

No matter how many times someone has tried to mold the value of confidence into your consciousness, because of its fragility, it's truly a trait that can't be reinforced enough. In order to be a high-performing individual, you must consistently recognize and appraise your levels of confidence across all facets of life. Whether it's an absence of appreciation for your appearance, low confidence in your ability to perform well in your career, or a shrinking reliance in a relationship, lacking assurance in any area will negatively affect your overall experience on Earth.

With that said, let's analyze how self-confidence is developed and how to properly maintain a positive attitude when thinking about your skills and abilities. In recent years, there's been a ton of studies published where, in each evaluation, researchers attempted to gain a better understanding of confidence as a whole. A plethora of studies backed up Deion Sanders, legendary member of the Pro Football Hall of Fame, who famously said, "If you look good, you feel good, and if you feel good, you play good," as numerous researchers proved that how you dress plays a lively role in your level of self-confidence. Not just what you put on, but even the color of your attire has been shown to influence degrees of self-belief.

One study by Northern University concluded that, if you wish to feel more driven and dominant, then you should habitually listen to music with a loud bassline. Researchers at the University of California, Irvine, found that snapping positive photos each day, like a picture of your smiling self or a portrait of something that makes you or another being happy can also aid in the boosting of self-confidence. Other beneficial actions include self-talk sessions (in which you say aloud positive affirmations), spending time with uplifting individuals, and positive self-reflection periods, either in thought or by way of journaling.

All of the aforementioned research is great, but the most important takeaway from the modern exploration of neuroplasticity is that human beings, no matter the age or energy expended in a particular area, always have the power to reprogram their brains and alter any belief that is not in alignment with their ideal self. It's simply a choice. If you choose to believe that you can tie your shoes, then that proves you have the ingrained strength to perceive anything as you please. The biochemistry of our body emanates from our core understanding of the truths in our reality, which, while following the laws of physics, is in our hands to interpret.

Aware of this, the question to ask is the following: What set of actions can a human take to ensure their self-belief levels are positioned in a strong enough zone that they are capable of energetically evolving into the optimal self?

From here, a being who wishes to increase confidence in a specific area must go through a process of "reasoning upwards" to identify the root of the potential issue. This means defining both the present-limiting and the future-fitting beliefs, then analyzing all of the concrete truths in relation to the affair. In the course of characterizing the present belief, it is imperative to train your brain to omit the negative thought, as it does no good for it to remain in your consciousness. If an individual presently lacks self-confidence in any space, they must avoid judging their effectiveness in it. If the negative belief lingers, it becomes increasingly more strenuous to alter it. Part of the reason why you're able to effortlessly tie your shoes is that the thought of not being able to is completely absent.

As basic as it sounds, this is how you must approach any mental obstacle. The only reason why the poor assumption was even present is because you chose to have it be. A belief gets stored in the brain through sources like our environment, past firsthand experiences, and knowledge in the area. Basically, what you've seen, heard, or been told shapes how you think. What you perceive to be true in mind becomes truth in reality, so the importance of removing all poor thoughts is apparent.

Once these steps are made, the person partaking in the exercise would follow it up with a series of efforts, either physical or mental, or both, that they must take to work toward the favored feeling. Through consistent work, it's only a matter of time before the ideal belief is a new, molded opinion.

Outside of facing the concern head-on, an individual who wishes to get a firm grasp on their ability to develop confidence in any desired area should seriously consider exercising because working out, as we know, enhances serotonin production, which, aside from its previously mentioned mental enrichments, also plays a crucial part in shaping our level of self-esteem. Researchers in this space associate high serotonin levels in the brain with high self-respect status, and low levels of the neurotransmitter with poor levels of self-confidence. This is primarily due to its tenacious ability to operate as a mood stabilizer. The stronger a grip one has on their emotions, the easier it is to process thought and productively move forward in any operation.

From a general perspective, the act of exercising involves a lively being who is taking action to improve both physical and mental health. This wise use of energy alone complements self-assurance because, at its core, the activity represents a human revving up their horsepower, which results in the priming of its corporal functionalities. Following an arduous workout, you can invariably say, with full conviction, that you used your stamina in a productive manner, improved your heart's health, got physically stronger, boosted mental aptitude, seized a better hold on your level of self-esteem, and immanently attained a sense of self-achievement. All of these cited realizations naturally put you in a winning situation.

Not to mention the most noticeable perk, which, of course, is explicit control over one's weight and overall bodily shape. To no surprise, carrying excess weight has been scientifically linked to one's state of mind. In one study in particular, published in the *Archives of General Psychiatry*, researchers found that adults in the experiment who carried excess weight had a 55 percent higher risk of developing depression over their existence than individuals who maintained a healthy BMI. Additional research also supports the idea that being overweight can lead to an increase in suffering from bipolar disorder and significant panic attacks.

Being overweight holds other possible consequences as well. Number one, a surplus of weight leads to chronic aches, which directly impacts mood. If a human is suffering from physical pain that was birthed because of their inability to maintain a healthy weight, then their quality of life immediately decreases, as they'll be unable to participate in actions that they enjoy with people who they love. An inactive social life can have a sizeable impact on our behavior patterns and typically translates to loneliness and extreme isolation, which generally forms feelings of depression. Aside from chronic soreness, concrete data has proven that being overweight increases inflammation. An escalation of inflammation has been linked to humans with considerable dispiritedness.

Us humans also have a natural "body bias" implanted in our consciousness that is sadly programmed to negatively characterize an obese individual. This abrogating perception is, of course, destructive to an overweight being's self-esteem and overall self-body image.

Outside of the serotonin found in the brain, the majority of our supply of the neurotransmitter, roughly 95 percent of it, is secreted in the gut. While the brain serotonin is an extreme plus, an inefficient use of the type found in your gut will increase blood glucose levels and fat mass, which, in turn, inflates the risk of obesity. Excess weight, in addition to its previously specified ramifications, has been shown to negatively impact hormone production, which can lower energy levels, thus producing an individual who, because of their body, will lack the desire to exercise and reap the otherworldly benefits.

One of the principal purposes of this part of the project was to emphasize the hulking, yet generally underestimated, impact that fitness has on the mind and the foundation of our beliefs. The quintessential, initial mental picture that a human visualizes when they hear the word "exercise" is an active, able-bodied being in the midst of a vigorous workout. While there's no denying the bodily benefits that are brought forth via a nice gym session, one could make a strong case that physical training does more for our brain than it does for our muscles. Its efficacious influences on thought, memory, and emotion alone make it arguably the most useful activity that one could put strength toward during their waking hours.

Again, all of these perks for the mind are naturally harvested just by breaking a sweat. You don't have to specialize in a particular fitness routine or thoughtfully train certain muscles. Just find a way to produce perspiration through your pores, and soak in the returns.

Looping in a leader who devotedly believed in the extreme power of exercising: in 1960, John F. Kennedy—American politician who served as the thirty-fifth president of the United States until his tragic assassination—authored an article for *Sports Illustrated*, titled "The Soft American." The president-elect, who grew up in a home that was dedicated to physical activity, penned the piece to promote the importance of physical fitness for Americans.

In the feature, Kennedy, a letter-winning swimmer at Harvard, directed his message particularly toward younger men, who he believed were presently not putting their best foot forward when it came to physical soundness. Early on in the think-piece, Kennedy wrote, "The first indication of a decline in the physical strength and ability of young Americans became apparent among

United States soldiers in the early stages of the Korean War." He then followed up this passionate jab with some startling statistics that proved the American youth was far behind the kids in Europe as far as physical fitness. "Six tests for muscular strength and flexibility were given," Kennedy reported. "57 percent of the American children failed one or more of these tests, while only 8.7 percent of the European youngsters failed."

Following additional use of data and a growing intensity in tone to further drive home his point, Kennedy, over sixty years ago, scripted a set of sentences that are in direct alignment with this very chapter. "For physical fitness is not only one of the most important key to a healthy body; it is the basis of dynamic and creative intellectual activity. The relationship between the soundness of the body and the activities of the mind is subtle and complex. Much is not yet understood. But we do know what the Greeks knew: that intelligence and skill can only function at the peak of their capacity when the body is healthy and strong; that hardy spirits and tough minds usually inhabit sound bodies."

When Kennedy says "what the Greeks knew," he's making reference to age-old thoughts that were hypothesized over 2,500 years ago by some of the greatest philosophers and caretakers in recorded human history. The ancient Greeks looked at physical fitness as somewhat of a national obligation for the members of their community, especially the young men, who were forcefully instructed to stay physically active in order to develop strength, discipline, and grit. This belief system was strikingly personified among the males in Sparta, a warrior society in ancient Greece. The Spartans, by way of a hard-nosed, state-sponsored education, military schooling, and socialization program, trained boys, beginning at the age of seven, to become the most courageous, patriotic, tenacious, and resilient soldiers of their time. These young men were directed to never show fear, or express emotion under any sort of pain, no matter the extremity of the injury. As many know, the Spartan society has been well-documented, as numerous literary works and motion pictures have been cultivated to distinctly depict the fictitious-sounding, savage-like civilization.

In addition to sharply sprouting a culture of valiant soldiers, the ancient Greeks are also famous for assembling the first Olympics in the summer of 776 BCE. The games were held in honor of Zeus, the Greeks' most esteemed and powerful god, at Olympia and included events like sprinting and wrestling, which are still part of today's modern games.

Not only did the populace comprehend the physical benefits birthed from working out, but the intellectual savants of the time were able to deeply analyze the culture and spot a clear, salubrious relationship between exercise and mental perspicacity.

The earliest recorded examples of Greek individuals using an open space as a gymnasium (plural *gymnasia*) date back to the sixth century BCE. Typically, the physical makeup of these training centers was a nice spot of land that was sheltered from the sun by trees and positioned near a body of rushing waters. It has been said that young Greek men (*ephebeia*) would be those primarily found here to physically train and prepare for warfare, but another belief is that these exercise fields were roped off for the aristocracy, as they would use the territory to enhance their physical and social skills far beyond those of the lower, agricultural class. Either way, the men in attendance were piercingly focused on improving their physical strength and hardening their minds.

According to the World History Encyclopedia, "the typical sports practiced were wrestling, running, boxing, jumping, discus, and gymnastics. Many would have been accompanied by rhythmic music. Sports useful for warfare included archery, javelin, armed combat, and using catapults." It is also believed that the nearby trees and rivers were used for climbing and swimming, respectively.

Whenever beings competed in any of the recreational activities, a trainer (*paidotribe*) would be in attendance to supervise the event. It is assumed that majority of these mentors were older athletes who clashed against top-tier opponents in previous years at the great Games of Greece. Identical to the genesis of the Olympics, the Greeks consistently held sporting games at these confines to honor their beloved heroes and gods. The contests, which often involved a torch race and a trio of other events that radiated vigor (*euexia*), discipline (*eutaxia*), and endurance (*philoponia*), quickly became a prominent part of the community's social life. The winner of one of these illustrious games was granted a wreath, and an abundant amount of honor and respect from his peers.

As time went on, the ancient Greek gyms evolved, starting from a place to exercise, train, and compete, to eventually incorporating aspects of education and health. Early on in their schooling process, young boys would spend a good chunk of their time at the gym, developing their strength, endurance, and war-ready mindset through physical exercise, but they were also schooled on the noteworthy benefits that come from maintaining a healthy body. Because of the instructive focus, it was incredibly common for philosophers to come and hold scholastic talks for the kids and any interested gatherers. Athens, in particular, had three storied gyms built at three acclaimed schools of philosophy: the Academy of Plato, Aristotle's Lyceum, and the Cynosarges, a famous temple of Heracles. This unification of intellectual education with physical fitness helped initiate some of the rationales provided in this very project.

Because of the society's Herculean focus on physical exercise and its ever-so-puissant relationship with the soul, distinguished ancient Greek philosophers and doctors made sure to document this uniquely strong correlation in notable ways. For example,

Pythagoras (570–490 BCE), ancient Ionian Greek philosopher and the eponymous founder of Pythagoreanism, was the first individual from ancient Greece to encourage daily exercise for health purposes. At the school he established in Croton, Italy, Pythagoras urged his adherents to stick to a regular routine of diet, exercise, music, and meditation if they wished to live a life of good health, inner harmony, and fulfilment.

Years later, Hippocrates (460–377 BCE), legendary Greek physician of the classical period, became the first recorded doctor to provide a scripted exercise remedy for a patient who was suffering from consumption. According to the article, "The History of 'Exercise Is Medicine' in Ancient Civilizations," published by the National Library of Medicine, Hippocrates "prescribed moderate exercise because it warned, thinned, and purged away the humor." (Humors were thought to include phlegm, yellow bile, black bile, and blood.) The author of the scholarly article went on to mention that "Hippocrates believed that training would increase stature, bone mass, muscle mass, tone, and endurance, digestion, temperature regulation, and tolerance against fatigue." Here are a pair of pertinent quotes (translated to Modern English), attributed to the "Father of Medicine" himself:

"Even when all is known, the care of a man is not yet complete, because eating alone will not keep a man well; he must also

take exercise. For food and exercise, while possessing opposite
qualities, yet work together to produce health."

"Walking is man's best medicine."

The aforementioned Plato, ancient Greek philosopher, once
stated, around 380 BCE, that "lack of activity destroys the
good condition of every human being, while movement and
methodical physical exercise save it and preserve it." (Modern
English translation)

In their own unique way, each of these esteemed individuals
overtly declared that a life without physical exercise is self-
sabotaging to the soul. What's interesting about Hippocrates's
first manifesto—which, by the way, is obviously up for debate as
to its exact connotation—is that he felt the need to specifically
mention how one can be a master in an area, but, if their
exercise and nutrition levels are not up to par, what they know
in this world immediately becomes less valuable, and more
fragile, since their physical and mental health are not being
properly commanded.

These assessments were made over two thousand years ago, yet
it feels as though the superannuated wisdom has been expunged
from the minds of the present mass. What's even sadder is that
Kennedy, over six decades ago, tried to reinforce these ancient
beliefs, speaking in spirited terms to educate the country on

the importance of physical fitness and its ever-so-prominent influence on quality of life, yet obesity rates and mental health issues continue to skyrocket.

On the bright side, the modern research that's been collected has allowed us to take what Hippocrates, Plato, and Kennedy postulated as undeniable truth and pair their logic with concrete science to make confident conclusions in this department. Up to this point in the project, we've discovered, through detailed examinations, that physical exercise has explicit effects on various sectors of the brain. These impressions pointedly support our memory, thought and emotional control, belief system, aptitude, decision-making, behaviors, energy level, and overall focus, to name a few.

In a compact recounting statement, consistent exercise enhances mental clarity, which allows us to have better control over our thoughts, feelings, and emotions. The stronger we feel, the easier it is to put energy toward an action that we wish to succeed in. The more control we have over our inner nature, the easier it becomes to make on-target decisions. Strong judgement, mixed with an effective action, blended with an unwavering belief, generates positive outcomes.

On the opposite end, lack of physical exercise will alter your ability to maintain a healthy weight. Inefficient weight management has been shown to noticeably alter our physical health, inner belief system, and overall state of mind, which is a recipe for disaster for those who wish to sustain greatness over the long run. To avoid cooking up this negative compound, one needs to work out and watch what they put inside their body.

In this realm, steady belief in oneself is a precursor to cogently connecting with the right individual, or group of people, who can radically help you reach your goals. With competition continuing to surge across all meaningful, well-respected careers, it is imperative that a soul, who wishes to excel, builds and nurtures the proper connections to give themselves, and their potential team, the strongest odds of victory. At the individual level, we possess an ample amount of strength and dynamism, but, when banded with other beings full of talent and might, we multiply our chances of embracing excellence. Recognizing this reality, the concept of networking becomes ever so necessary to grasp. To be frank, our level of self-belief, whether it be in who we are as a person, or in our ideas, will directly determine our effectiveness in uniting. If you are seeking advice from a master in a field that you wish to grow in, the expert in the situation would naturally be more willing to aid you if they recognized a strong level of self-confidence, as this gives them a reason to dedicate time and energy toward you and your endeavor. Deep down, humans want to assist and collaborate with those who express profound passion, candid curiosity, and steadfast self-assurance, as this amalgamation of attributes tellingly shows another being that you have the proper makeup for advancement.

This holds true for associating with a coach, business partner, friend, lover, coworker, teacher, potential client, or even family member. The more self-assurance we radiate, the more we bring to the table in any relationship or social interaction.

One of the biggest factors in making a strong first impression with a person is self-courage status. If we come across as weak, or timid in our personal attributes and intellectual sense, then we create a massive barrier between where we presently stand in the relationship and what's potentially possible. Luckily, just by staying physically active, you instinctively halt the possible feelings of weakness that could otherwise have been expressed, had your brain not been operating at full capacity or your body not been where you wanted it.

While this may feel minuscule and unimportant to the intention of this book, the fact of the matter is this: We aren't on this journey alone, and, if we wish to maximize our time and actualize all of our aspirations, then we need to effectively communicate with each other. Opportunities in this life come to those who are both mentally and physically ready to clutch the challenge and rise to the occasion. If you don't have your beliefs in check, and your mental clarity isn't on point, then the moment will not hesitate to pass you by. Whether it be a profitable business venture, potent relationship, or personal event in your arena that can elevate your worth, the universe will give you what you can

perceptually spot, and ultimately what you think you deserve
to receive.

The most practical piece of advice to offer someone who wishes
to consistently find themselves in, and ready for, promising
opportunities, is to tell them to immediately start being the
person that they desire to be. All of us are dreamers at heart, and,
as sensible souls, we have a superbly rare ability to discreetly draw
up mental scenes in our mind that can corporeally adjust our
emotional state. Just by visualizing yourself in an uplifting act,
your body can sense the scenario as if it was physically playing out
in the three-dimensional reality, which is quite uncanny when
you really think about it.

Anyways, when positive pictures are produced in the mind, the
portrait usually presents the fantasizer at the pinnacle of their
favored field, with their desired partner, amongst their cherished
friends, surrounded by their kids, or even in their dream car.
No matter the specifics of the plot, when a forward-looking
image involving the individual is created, the main entity in the
sight is always in a peak state of being. Knowing the ultimate
objective is to be the person in our minds who generated the
feel-good state, the obvious step to take for physical realization
would be to reverse-engineer the process, so that, in due time,
we morph into our top-notch self. To begin this procedure, we
must first examine our apex character. Then, we must instantly
adopt the traits and features of our ideal. Physically, how is the

quintessential self shaped? How does the being dress? Who
does this individual spend time around? What does this person
put energy toward during their waking hours? How do they
communicate with others? What activities are they part of that
feed their soul? What are their passions? How do they walk, and,
in times of rest, how do they sit? Do they favor an upright seated
posture, as opposed to a slouching stance, to enhance their mood,
rate of speech, and concentration? (Research shows that specific
muscular and autonomic states have the power to impact our
emotions and our ability to effectively focus.) How do they think?
How are they making a living, and what did they do to earn a
strong level of respect from their peers?

These are all standard questions that one should ask themselves
as they start to progress toward the superlative self. Once these
inquiries are clearly answered, the next step would be to make
the necessary changes in your present existence to ensure that
you put yourself in a perfect position to become the emblematic
person that you know you are capable of becoming. Since
the image of the fitting character was already seen and felt in
the mind, this means that transforming into that person is a
legitimate possibility in reality. Understanding this, once the
alterations are made, meaning the habits and thoughts are now
directly in line with the way the ideal operates, it's only a matter
of time before the present soul and paradisiacal being merge into
one. Simply put, if you act and perform as the ideal acts, then, by
definition, you *are* the ideal.

Living in the end, and scrupulously studying the exemplary self, is essential for personal fulfillment because the positive portraits that you metaphorically paint in your mind are the visions that your inner being wishes to materialize the most. Since the feelings of happiness are generated from within, your fantasies as a daydreamer are the spectacles that your soul deems the most gratifying and wondrous outcomes to play out in reality.

This all ties in with fitness because the enhancement in mental lucidity that is emanated from working out directly impacts a human's ability to analyze internally. The more we exercise, the clearer we think. The clearer we think, the easier it is to conceptualize our true desires. By tightly gripping and verily sensing our aspirations, we naturally increase our odds of creating whatever it is that we strive for.

Although we briefly touched on the shoe thesis earlier in this section, as a necessary reminder, a principal reason as to why you're able to successfully lace up your shoes is because you carry an unshakeable belief in your ability to execute the act. All individuals are unable to consistently achieve the appropriate result when they first start trying to tie their shoes because their confidence in their talent resides on the ground floor. It is practically nonexistent. Aware of this, one should immediately recognize strong self-belief as a fundamental precursor to attainment in any area.

In addition, as part of symbolically stamping a strong level of self-confidence onto your soul so that you're well-equipped to fulfil any objective, make sure that your degree of personal belief comes with full detachment from the ideal outcome. In other words, you are so certain of your ability to create the right result that spending time analyzing how you might, or might not, reach the finish line isn't even remotely a consideration. When you attempt to tie your shoes, in the midst of the act, you most likely do not internally say to yourself, "I need to be able to tie my shoes," or, "I don't know if I can tie my shoes," or even, "The goal is to tie my shoes and I must complete it." Because of the level of certainty that you have in your ability to produce the proper reaction, you're able to metaphorically "stay out of your own way," allowing you to easily succeed in the act. Your brain knows that you want to tie your shoes, you undoubtedly believe in your ability to perform, and then you put energy toward the feat and make it happen.

When you second-guess your power to create favorable results in your reality, you immediately confuse your mind by consciously cultivating alternative options other than the optimal one. For some odd reason, as our aims in life become larger and more complex (on paper), the majority of humans tend to become more susceptible to doubting their ability to achieve the sought-after goal, which emphatically hurts their chance to succeed. Remember, the only way an aspiration could appear "loftier" or "harder to reach" is because of a preconceived notion that you may have mustered up in your mind. As a conscious being, you're the one who applies the level of difficulty to everything that you go after. For the best results, the same level of self-confidence that you have in your ability to tie your shoes should be figuratively carried into all of your other desired objectives, because triumphantly lacing up your kicks is no different than accomplishing anything else in this space. With your shoes, you picked out a goal in the three-dimensional world, and, by following the recipe for success, you achieved what you set out to. That right there is exactly what we aspire to do across all areas of our lives, so why would we alter a formula that has been proven to work to perfection? No matter what you aspire to, simply plant the treasured result in your brain, completely disconnect from whether or not it will come true, and stick by the blueprint for achievement.

Speaking of the previously penned compound for success, our belief system influences all four of the elements. In order to "own the appropriate resources," your mind has to be as sharp as a knife, and actively aware of what's needed for clear achievement. This could mean recruiting the right individuals around you to support an idea, or independently making alterations when it comes to your present pursuit.

Much like the intelligence chapter, "having a clear understanding of the outcome" is only possible when gazing through the brightest lens. This implies putting yourself in the right position for success by constantly rectifying your mental attitude. Outside of energy put toward the literal act, this can be reached by habitually working up a sweat by way of a physical drill.

Rule number three, "Take consistent action to further improve your success rate when performing the act," is applicable here because the effectiveness of the refinements you make with each proceeding move is directly related to how well you can examine the scene. Your level of understanding of how to excel in any area is the difference between succeeding and failing, so knowing how to properly analyze outcomes becomes ever-so-vital.

Most prominent in this part was the final rule. As previously emphasized, all individuals in this sphere have the ability to control their level of self-belief in whatever they put mental thought toward. Carrying an unshakeable belief in your ability to flourish in the desired feat is a choice—a decision that all should choose to make. If you've been given the gift to exist in the flesh, and are aiming to maximize your physical efforts, you must believe that you can excel in whatever you choose to do. Rogers Hornsby, statistically one of the greatest hitters in MLB history, was once asked in an interview how he felt about the opposing pitchers that he had to face each time he stepped into the batter's box. The ballplayer, whose .358 career batting average stands as the second-highest mark in MLB history, answered by saying, "The only emotion or thought I ever had for a pitcher was to feel sorry for him. Maybe that's why I could hit." In other words,

whether you're competing against yourself, or clashing with
an opponent, stably believe that you are the greatest, and that
nothing in this world can get in the way of you accomplishing
whatever it is that you set out to.

Whether you are cognizant of it or not, your perception of self is
steadily, yet somewhat stealthily, altering, and this subtle shift is
strongly dependent on the specifics within the environment that
you're presently existing in. How you recognize yourself is tied to
your past recollection, plus your current conditions, which means
you are essentially a completely different person depending
on the nature of your present surroundings, and the previous
information you elect to focus your attention on in real time.
This assessment holds a strong level of accuracy in a social circle,
where, as humans, we will naturally rank ourselves somewhere
amongst the herd, and reach a conclusion that is comprised
of prior interactions and past analysis, mixed in with current
observations. In reference to "prior interactions," depending on
the status of your emotional strength, any energy, whether it be
positive or negative, that gets pointedly thrown at you by way of
another human being has the potential to resolutely reshape your
self-belief state.

This theory also holds true in a competitive space, where we will
inherently estimate the stature of our skills in comparison to the
field, and place ourselves somewhere amongst the bunch in terms
of talent level. Even in times when we find ourselves alone, we

will innately stick a value on our head that's calculated from our present self-belief status. For a harmonious and prolific life, we must always be aware of this camouflaged calculation, and train our minds to automatically remain confident in our thoughts, demeanor, and abilities, no matter the technicalities of the scene. Never mind the room you're in, who you're speaking to, your relationship with the action that you're presently putting energy toward, or what you choose to recall about yourself from the past. Always make a deliberate effort to perpetually parade the planet with puissance.

In the song "Doo Wop (That Thing)," which is arguably the most commemorated track from Lauryn Hill's hallowed album, *The Miseducation of Lauryn Hill*, the gracious artist, nearing the end of her second verse, eloquently asks the listener, "How you gon' win when you ain't right within?" She then proceeds to repeat the inquiry two more times before working to the bridge of her anthem.

Whenever I am at a standstill with a particular obstacle, or question my inherent strength, I think about Ms. Hill's line, and remind myself that achieving greatness is downright impossible without a proper mindset. Reaching true eminence requires years and years of consistent and outstanding output. Preeminent production is propagated by people who possess prodigious packs of power. Power in body, and power in mind.

Aside from pervading doughty dynamism, all bona fide champions employ a specific way of reasoning to attack their aims. It's something called "target-based thinking," which is the appellation for the next phase of the project, and a compelling reasoning method that is hyper-inveigled through fitness.

Chapter 4

TARGET-BASED THINKING

There's an axiological reason why having a distinct understanding of the optimal target is one of our four ingredients for true attainment. Without identifying an X on our map of desired objectives, the toilsome path on the road to remarkable achievement is rather meaningless. Simply put, by not setting purposeful goals, humans jeopardize their ability to positively influence their surroundings and, most tragically, limit their personal output. I consider hindering your individual production level to be dreadful because, in this experience, we are regularly remembered only by our actions and words. If you don't have clear-cut aims behind your efforts, you directly bruise your own legacy.

The mere act of establishing an aspiration forces any and all beings to put time and energy toward manufacturing a particular outcome. Manifesting positive results is a prerequisite to classifying someone as a successful human being. Think about all the individuals you consider to be "influential" or "well-off." While everyone is different, one constant that will always remain amongst prosperous people is that they all consistently hit impressive targets. These desires vary depending on career path, but, regardless of the uniqueness in the intention, flourishing individuals routinely set marks and find ways to reach them. The most impactful people are genuinely just the ones who fulfill the most appreciated and/or arduous ambitions.

A life without goals is a directionless one. Feelings on the lower end of the emotional spectrum, like stress, anxiousness, sadness, concern, and discomfort, are forcibly amplified in negative fashion when a lack of direction is present. When felt, these poor feelings prohibit progress.

Comprehending this, an educated approach to bypass feeling desultory would be to ensure that we consistently, and clearly, classify specific targets for whatever we decide to put stamina toward. Identical to spotting the supreme self, when an ultimate end for any of one's ambitions is identified, the level of certainty in their ability to successfully perform the act will inevitably increase. The clearer the vision of the desired end result, the easier it is to recognize how to go about attaining the aim.

This method of thinking has been echoed throughout this entire book. However, the reasoning behind emphasizing the importance of labeling a destination point is not just for repetition purposes. Its noted intent for this chapter is to illustrate how a standard exercise routine involves an array of objectives, which instinctively supports your everyday thinking patterns and forces you to adopt a target-based mindset.

Common exercise activities, like walking, running, biking, strength training, circuit training, swimming, and playing sports, all involve numerical systems to track an individual's progress. For all of the listed aerobic workouts, a person determines their level of skill in the particular pursuit by measuring their speed and distance. This could mean a sprinter calibrating how fast they can run a certain stretch or a swimmer calculating how many meters they can swim in a particular amount of time. In the weight room, it is popular to track how many pounds you can lift in a desired drill, and/or how many reps you can successfully complete of a physical act. As many know, sports, especially at the professional level, are flooded with statistics to help record performance.

What's interesting about humans, from a pure science perspective, is that they'll always yearn for more. The drive to seek out more has been commonly considered as the most-generated primary instinct in the human brain. Even the most accomplished individual in this experience will always feel the need to explore further. No one will ever really feel as though they've "made it" or that they've "checked off all the boxes," There will always be a new desire ahead.

The aforementioned neurotransmitter, dopamine, in addition to its previously-touched-on benefits, also causes humans to want, crave, hunt, and search for more. A mental and emotional uptick in appetite in any area directly influences a human's behavior—so much so that the dopamine kick you receive from partaking in a pleasing, positive activity will inherently force you to take additional action toward said activity in the hopes of mirroring the sensation of reward felt from the release of the neurotransmitter. The deep-seated force can also be simply thought of as love. When you are enamored by someone or something, dopamine, norepinephrine, and serotonin are the neurotransmitters that actually father the feeling of attraction. The more infatuated we are with another being or a particular activity, the higher our dopamine levels will be.

This is why people who are passionate and proficient in particular hobbies are always naturally seeking to improve and learn more about their field. No one needs to tell a young, enthusiastic basketball player to go shoot hoops or encourage a guitar aficionado to practice his shredding skills. The ingrained love for the activity, mixed with the gratification sensed from succeeding in the act, creates the dopamine release which forces both the athlete and musician to continually spend time in their specific craft.

Obviously, because of its active role in how we sense drive and affection, dopamine can be somewhat of a double-edged sword. In this sphere, not everything we are attracted to or in love with is of benefit for personal output, so, in order to accurately observe the healthiness in someone's levels of dopamine, one must ensure that the boost of the neurotransmitter is a direct reaction from being around positive people or partaking in a pursuit that is profitable for personal production.

For the purpose of this project, this substance is relevant because, as we know, the brain releases a great deal of dopamine when we are physically active. This discharge positively remodels our mind, and if we habitually exercise, the brain will actually show an expansion in dopamine receptor availability. This was effectively highlighted in a 2008 study titled "Neuroplasticity of Dopamine Circuits After Exercise: Implications for Central Fatigue." The authors, Monika Fleshner and Teresa E Foley, conducted various animal studies and concluded that aerobic exercise has the power to increase dopamine levels in the striatum, hypothalamus, midbrain, and brain stem. Below is a brief outline of the four noted regions and their vital functions:

- **Striatum:** Involves neuronal activity associated with movements and *rewards*.
- **Hypothalamus:** Helps keep the body in a calm state known as homeostasis.
- **Midbrain:** Aids with motor movement, specific motion of the eye, and auditory and visual processing.
- **Brain stem:** Supports breathing, consciousness, heart rate, and sleep.

Because the striatum plays such a significant role in reward processing, the dopamine boost in this region that is supplied from regularly exercising means that our brains will literally become more receptive to joy and enhance the capacity to sense the actual sensation felt from all fruitful experiences.

This is why it is incredibly common for cardio fans to feel an immediate sense of bliss following an effortful run. This "runner's high," as many refer to it, is felt because, when you move at a high speed, a rush of endorphins bind to receptors of the central nervous system. When this happens, dopamine is released, which promptly creates the sense of elation.

Additionally, when one participates in a physical workout, their brain produces a surplus of oxytocin in the hypothalamus. For those unaware, oxytocin is commonly referred to as the "love hormone," as it helps us connect on a deeper level with who and what we love.

Now, getting back to the relationship between exercising and goal setting and why it's all of benefit for your day-to-day operations. As mentioned, essentially all popular forms of physical exercise provide a strong amount of clarity to mark performance. Enhanced visibility in any field naturally encourages humans to aspire for self-improvement. Knowing that you can do thirty pull-ups in a row or that you can run a mile in under six minutes is the type of data that gets planted in your brain and is used as motivation for the next time you put energy toward these exercises.

This concept is also relevant for those who work out to lose weight. Just by recognizing your present number on the scale, you possess an inherent motivation to shed as many pounds as necessary. Each time you measure your weight and see an improvement, the natural desire to continue working expands. When you possess the passion to progress in the fitness space, you will instinctively find yourself setting aims to hit in future workouts. This could mean trimming down to a specific weight by a particular date or being able to perform a definite number of push-ups in any given set.

Since exercising is a gainful activity for both body and mind, the more we do it, the more likely it is that we will push to improve. As mentioned, the increase in dopamine that is supplied from working out scientifically allows for an enhancement in how we sense reward. When a comfortable amount of joy is perceived in any satisfying act, humans are more likely to put additional time and energy into said activity. A surge in stamina spent in any space primarily leads to an uptick of arranged intentions in the area. In other words, we are more prone to set goals and work hard to fulfill them when our declared aims are incorporated with activities that we love. Not only are we more likely to establish targets in fields that we adore, but, the deeper the reverence, the higher we will shoot for greatness.

Science backs this up. Research has shown that people with high levels of dopamine will actually work harder to attain a greater goal, and enjoy a larger reward, than those with low levels of the noted neurotransmitter, who, in experiments, were more likely to take the easy road and receive a smaller honor.

A strong eagerness to elevate, potently blended with a deep sense of adoration, mixed with a clear-cut aim, is a recipe for sweeping success. Top this formula off by consistently maintaining high dopamine levels, and you've now programmed your body and mind to become a powerful performer. As penned earlier, high-performers are merely individuals who customarily accomplish lofty goals. Once you make it a habit to routinely exercise, the enriched visibility into individual production levels, fused with the provided mental sparks, inherently influences your mind to constantly set targets and work hard to recognize them—thus putting you in a fantastic position to become a legendary figure.

So what actually happens in our minds when we set targets? Before that question is directly answered, let's begin from the basement by quickly defining what exactly a "target" is. In this case, a target is any desired result that wouldn't otherwise materialize without some form of intervention. Whenever one is set, there is an imaginary bridge: on one side lies the present reality, and the other is home to a world in which the aim is fully realized. In order to move across the bridge with the hopes of properly manifesting the ideal outcome, there must be a strong sense of motivation present. In other words, an unwavering desire to accomplish the aim serves as the energy needed to get from A to B. Without the inclination to achieve, the bridge cannot be crossed.

When a definitive target is specified, either in mind or seeded in the sphere via written word or by speaking aloud, the particular aim is given reward value in the brain. From there, dopamine is released, which creates the mental impulse to fulfill the ambition. The higher the value we place on the target, the more potent the dopamine surge.

It should be noted that there have been studies published in which researchers found that individuals who scripted their aims were actually more likely to accomplish their stated desires than those who opted to keep their individual targets within their minds. Whether you believe in the power of the written word or not, as long as you firmly retain the objective in any manner, your mind will operate accordingly.

This dopamine kick you get from setting goals essentially serves as a reminder-flag in your mind or, in the above example, the other end of the bridge. Understanding that the only barrier between our current state and a reality featuring the obtained objective is the drive to take the necessary action, an obvious thought would be to understand how a sense of motivation can be actively felt and maintained throughout the journey. The more alive your engine is, the easier it is to create your ideal reality.

To further decipher the roots of inner drive, we must first have an understanding of the factors that directly impact an individual's motivation levels. Unfortunately, the determinants that influence desire are solely dependent on the specific objective that one is presently focused on. Your physiological and psychological states, environment, and past history all have a hand in how ambitious you are in a particular scenario. Depending on the details of the scene, their levels of influence can vary greatly.

In addition to the three referenced factors, the relationship between the costs and rewards that spawn from putting energy toward the goal matters greatly—costs meaning time, effort, and sacrifices, and possible pain in the pursuit, versus the gratifying rewards that could be sensed when everything materializes. If the price to achieve the aim significantly outweighs the benefit from it, then it would obviously be difficult to remain driven throughout the process. On the other end, when a goal with a high reward is established, individuals are considerably more likely to push through the potential obstacles in order to reap the benefits.

With that said, it's clear that motivation can only be accurately assessed on a case-by-case basis. Determining this from an overarching perspective, before even zoning in on your goals, individuals need to ensure that they are in a strong position to effectively focus energy into an intention. This involves maintaining sharp levels of awareness, focus, self-belief, physical vigor, and mental acuity—all states that, as we've learned, are emphatically nourished through physical exercise.

Once these itemized elements are habitually sustained at a healthy level, the focus can now shift to desire, which, as we've come to find, is heavily influenced by our dopamine levels. Recognizing this, all individuals who aspire to regularly realize their aims should make it a daily priority to take the actions necessary that will naturally increase levels of dopamine. Since partaking in aerobic exercise, preferably for at least twenty minutes, has been scientifically shown to boost levels of the monoamine neurotransmitter across multiple sectors in the brain, one could confidently surmise that physical exercise is a perfect program to enhance levels of goal-setting and goal-achieving.

It's also worth pointing out that there are a handful of other actions, aside from physical fitness, that one can partake in to naturally elevate their dopamine levels. Eating foods that are rich in protein, getting an adequate amount of sleep each night, jamming out to some music, meditating, and spending time in the sun, have all been backed by science as effective ways to organically boost dopamine. Yet, because of the major effects that daily exercise has on both body and mind, many would argue that working out is the most influential act when it comes to raising our "feel-good" neurotransmitter.

In life, in order to reach great heights, we must set goals that supply us with a strong sense of gratification, and, simultaneously, ones that, when fulfilled, are universally recognized as tremendous achievements. However, before even focusing on getting to the top of the mountain, you must ensure that your infrastructure is as solid as a rock. In this sense, I am speaking of one's foundation for setting intentions. In order to perform as, and morph into, your ideal self, you must establish daily aims to train your mind to invariably think objectively. Without organizing targets to hit, you intentionally neglect the drive-magnifier that is activated by the dopamine release. In basic terms, if you choose to not set marks, your mind will not receive any signals to prompt your body into taking action toward achievement. This, in turn, will directly reduce the potency of your superpowers.

Along with the many cited perks that come from habitually exercising, one of its truly undervalued benefits is its remarkable influence on our competitive juices. Let's face it, whether you're running, lifting weights, or circuit training, performing any high-intensity workout is not easy. Within any legitimate exercise activity, you are pushing your body beyond its comfort zone and, in extreme cases for seasoned athletes, seeing how far you can take it before failure. If effectively exercising on a consistent basis was a walk in a park, the world wouldn't have so many nations that are flooded with overweight individuals.

With all that said, its level of difficulty is invaluable, because it's what generates the mighty dopamine release. A highly strenuous workout fuels us with the most power because, internally, the harder the mission, the deeper we sense the reward when the task is completed. Take a step back and ruminate over some of the past moments in your life in which you pushed beyond your preconceived limits to reach a destination point. Chances are, these memories, once the target was hit, are the ones that provided you with the highest amount of joy.

For the gamers out there, if you were a building a video game character, and your goal was to make the being as close to a superhero as possible, the number one action you would take to ensure their internal drive, physical build, and mental keenness was maxed out would be putting the creation through an intensified drill of any kind. Knowing this, the only thing stopping you in the real world from becoming your champion-self is a lack of energy put toward extreme physical and mental activities. In this astonishing reality, it is entirely possible to transform yourself into a real-life superhero, but reaching this prestige requires a protracted trek down the path of most resistance, which involves a lifelong, competitive battle against the being that you see in the mirror.

To compete is to deliberately drive for a particular objective. In common competition, people strive for various aims, such as a prize, like a team trophy or personal award, a status position, or a specific profit amount. In any competitive space, contestants in the arena are forced to bring out the best version of themselves, as anything less could lamentably result in a lack of success.

The act of physical competition is best expressed through sports. At the pro level, a sea of spirited spectators, in any given event, witness the most talented athletes at their craft going head-to-head with each other with the hopes of winning the explicit battle. What's beautiful about athletics is that, in most matches, only one player, or team, depending on the specifics of the bout, gets crowned. There is a winner, and there's a loser. No in-between.

To reach the top in any athletic field, one must spend countless hours honing their craft, while simultaneously making gobs of sacrifices along the way. For the rare breeds that do arrive at the pinnacle, becoming the 1 percent of the 1 percent, the stakes are now the highest, from both a competitive and financial standpoint; individual and team legacies are on the line, and personal pride is at its apex. Millions of fans, ranging from young kids to grown adults, religiously tune in to support their efforts and excitedly watch them perform.

This compelling compound of elements cultivates an environment of heightened competition. The level of difficulty in the game is why you see so many professional players get emotional following a winner-take-all event. The victorious ones cry tears of joy, as they mentally recall how much hard work and dedication was put into their successful efforts. On the other end, despite potentially mirroring the drive of the triumphant ones, those who were unable to execute in timely fashion sob in sadness, knowing they will have to report back to the lab and make adjustments for the next time around.

This is why the product of professional sport is so lucrative. Within the field of play lie some of the most determined beings the world has ever seen, who, for a good chunk of their existence on Earth, pushed, and continue to drive themselves, beyond physical and mental boundaries to earn their spot. The best of the best, squaring off in physical fashion for one goal. A recipe that has had the masses glued to the games since the contests were created.

A pair of recent examples of remarkable showdowns in team sports includes LeBron James and the Cleveland Cavaliers storming back from a 3–1 series deficit in the 2016 NBA Finals to astoundingly defeat the mighty, seventy-three-win Golden State Warriors, and the 2004 Boston Red Sox, en route to winning their first World Series Championship since 1918, shockingly swarming back against the powerhouse New York Yankees in the American League Championship Series after dropping the first three games.

Because of the aforementioned elements that coincide with performing at the top level, the intense competition created an atmosphere in which the participants, comprehending the significance of the reward, received a potent release of dopamine, which inherently served as a personal energy boost throughout the action. In both scenarios, the prizewinning players, as a collective, possessed a heightened level of focus, intense drive, and strong mental clarity, which allowed them to successfully obtain the objective. These two cases are great because, right before the Cavaliers and Red Sox flipped the script and charged back against their opponents, the odds of achieving their goal was so low, yet the two squads were able to keep the faith and prevail. If you ever feel down and out, think about these teams. Prior to their epic performances, in the history of the NBA, no team had ever dug themselves out of a 3–1 hole in the Finals. In MLB, no squad had ever abolished a 3–0 deficit in a seven-game series. Translation: Even when you feel buried deep down in the trenches, never give up.

Outside of sports, and any other standardized game, the spirit of competition is active across an array of areas that involve successful ventures. If you're creating a valuable product or service, you're most likely going up against hundreds, possibly thousands, of other individuals that are attempting to accomplish the same aim, and are doing everything they can to steal your potential customers. If you're in a creative arts field, like music, painting, acting, or writing, each day you put energy toward your craft, you must live with the fact that there are countless other beings who are readily battling against you to ensure they command the spotlight in the desired field.

With that said, in addition to frequently hitting worthwhile targets, successful people in this reality are those who are able to effectively outcompete the opposition. Knowing this, if you aspire to become the best version of yourself, you must master the art of competing against others, and, most importantly, the soul in the mirror.

Before even looping in the scientific facts around the mind, competition, and exercising, let's analyze the physical and mental battle that takes place each time you participate in a vigorous workout. At its core, to exercise is to actively engage in physical activity with the hope of enhancing health and fitness. Within any given physical drill, you are instructing your body to embrace a temporary sensation of somatic soreness in order to ultimately grow. The soreness spawns because, during a spirited session, you stress your muscles and the fibers start to break down. Fortunately, as the fibers mend themselves, they immediately become weightier and stronger than they were before.

From a mental vantage point, whenever you move around some weight, perform a sit-up, or take a sound stride amid a severe sprint, your mind is telling your body to negate its preconceived principles for a greater purpose. The idea of straining your muscles goes against our inherent code, as our bodies are naturally constructed to ensure that we exist in a pain-free state. This idea is easily illustrated through a possible outcome that could occur while one is in the middle of cooking. Let's say you're in the kitchen chopping up some garlic, and all of a sudden, you accidentally slice your pinky with a knife. The moment after cutting your finger, by way of magic, your body instantaneously begins to repair the wound. This example, along with our muscles getting bigger after breaking down, shows us that, without putting thought toward anything, we are existing in a build that is equipped with supernatural powers.

Perceiving this, it's clear that the act of physically exercising formulates a highly competitive battle against your own mind. When you're tired in the middle of a run or feel like putting the dumbbells down midway through a set because the shaky sensation in your arms is potently sensed, the choice to keep going results in an internal victory. Not only does the continuation of the challenging act benefit you from a physical standpoint, but mentally, it formally teaches the mind to push through pain while striving for a target. These specific acts of perseverance, when consistently engaged in, will help mold your warrior mentality, which, in turn, directly assists with how you take on any day-to-day objective.

Now, to briefly tie in some brain science. In a 2020 study funded by the National Natural Science Foundation of China, a research team was interested in exploring the attractive idea of aerobic exercise as a practical action to take to mitigate mood symptoms. In their experiment, the investigators gathered up a group of twelve- to fourteen-year-olds who reported having depressive and/or manic feelings. For the test, the kids, who were pulled from a middle school in Guangzhou, China, underwent an exercise program in which they would run for thirty minutes a session, four days a week, for three months. Following evaluation, which included a set of MRI scans, the research squad found that the cardio drill had a direct impact on the participants' anterior cingulate cortex (ACC), a major brain region that concerns mood control, emotion expression, and attention allocation. More specifically, the analysis showed that a troop of students, after habitually running for a few months, actually had increased structural volume in their left rostral ACC and enhanced cortical thickness in their right rostral ACC. This is influential because previous studies have found that weakened structural volume in the ACC can correlate with bipolar feelings.

What's even more interesting about the ACC is that, in a separate study, Dr. Kirstin Hillman and Professor David Bilkey from the Department of Psychology of the University of Otago (New Zealand), evaluated a group of free-roaming rats as they acted in a competitive drill that the intellects set up. In the operation, the rodents battled for a finite amount of food. In order to receive the grub, the rats had two options: move along an unimpeded path to reap a small reward, or head down a challenging track that came with a larger prize. In the middle of the action, the researchers tracked the activity in the rats' ACCs. The results revealed that, while the rats competed, neurons in the ACC were readily active. In addition, the activeness of the cells was completely independent of the outcome, meaning that, no matter which option the rats took, the sheer fact that they were competing for a select amount of food was enough to trigger the ACC.

In real time, the rats comprehended what was at stake, made a decision that would directly influence the outcome, and then competed with each other with the hopes of manifesting their desired result. This of course makes sense, as attention allocation has previously been paired with this region in the animal brain. However, knowing that the actual size of the ACC can be impacted through physical fitness, one could assuredly assume that working out is an incredibly effective action to take to further heighten your focus in times of competition.

Again, this information is rather pertinent to the purpose of the project because, no matter what anyone says, we all strive to live a happy and successful life. Focusing on the latter want, the fortunate humans are the ones who habitually hit targets and steadily stomp their competitors. To be mentioned amongst the fruitful fellows, you must do both. By happy chance, consistently exercising has a prominent effect on your eagerness to set aims and effectively compete. Without even eyeballing the science piece, anyone who has ever participated in a workout can understand the competitive value within the action. By physically pushing your body, you send a message to your inner being which states that you're willing to battle with the interim discomfort for a greater cause. This act alone boosts your competitive might like no other, which, in turn, raises your innate drive to attack any worthwhile objective.

On the flip side, if you lack competitive spirit and elect to saunter through life with no definitive direction, you'll be unable to productively perform in the present moment. The "now" is all we have, so your energy and your level of focus are the only two factors that you can tangibly control in the present. In layman's terms, to not set targets is to not prepare, and if you're equipped with a shortage of fighting force, you can pretty much guarantee that your inherent superhero abilities will never see the light of day. To make matters worse, when we neglect the idea of internally imprinting intentions, the above-mentioned idea of longing to live a joyous and lucrative life becomes next to impossible. By way of an allegorical address, an archer can have a crisp set of arrows and an adequate bow, but if there is no target set for him to shoot at, his weapons are of no value. When one's spirit lacks worth, their active energy within is drained, which then causes a clear collapse in concentration. If this combination is wrongfully activated by any being with senses, they are more than likely plunging down a path of darkness and defeat, which, from a pure mental health standpoint, is why it's so important to identity a purpose and routinely push toward it with your native zip.

Just being cognizant of the fact that your body is omnipotent should gift you with enough awareness and motivation to have the drive to consistently nurture your strength in a proper manner, yet so many individuals in this sphere overlook their immeasurable power. This is because, as modern humans, we unintentionally, but also sometimes willfully, cloud our path with so many distractions that most people end up simply accepting who they have been told they are, and what social class they belong in. Since you are reading this as a boundless being, this way of thinking is completely pointless, and the only thing stopping you from becoming a storied figure is a refusal to trek down a challenging trail with a clear target, and a determined spirit.

Succinctly looping in the Shoe Theory, the act of successfully lacing up your kicks is on the easier end mainly because the objective in the operation is clear-cut. You know exactly why you're putting energy toward the deed, which allows you to mentally picture the entire process from the finish line.

When a goal is consistently marked, and unceasingly envisioned in mind, you stick to it like a magnet, and, by way of magic, become energetically attracted to it. This principle holds true for all of your fixed aspirations, no matter the preconceived level of difficulty. Knowing this, it only makes sense to set the loftiest aims because, internally, once any objective is established, whether it's tying your shoes or creating a billion-dollar business, your brain goes to work for you. The cultivated coercive pull inherently constructs a path of success and immanently forces you to take the necessary set of actions that will naturally allow the aim to fully materialize in reality. The timing of the manifestation is solely dependent on your inherent drive and ability to follow the recipe for successful realization.

Speaking of the formula for achieving any goal, this section in the story, as previously mentioned, was obviously constructed around the second rule, which is "Have a clear understanding of the ideal outcome." It is impossible to achieve anything if the "thing" is not defined. While remaining on a clear, objective-marked course sounds smooth and overt, unfortunately, because of the way this experience is constructed, all beings are easily capable of drifting off the path. A key way to avoid sliding off the street to success is by making your personal aims a top priority. This can be done by constantly reviewing them each morning, either in mental thought, on paper, or aloud to yourself. However you choose to recall your ambitions, make sure they are actively imagined and vividly sensed. The more you focus on them, the stronger the gravitational pull, which is another way of saying, increased time spent concentrating on your goals leads to a direct enhancement in desire and inherent motivation to accomplish them. Interestingly enough, the more devoted you become to attaining your objectives, the worse you will feel in times when you slack off, which, in turn, strongly steers you back toward your purpose. This is something called "going against the aim" (not to be confused with the phrase *go against the grain*). When intentions are passionately set, anytime you waste energy in areas that do not align with your desired destination point, you will staunchly sense a feeling that corresponds with "misuse of time," which creates an inner craving to go even harder toward your marks. So don't just set goals to set goals. Fondly map out missions that are as lucid as Nas's lyrics on *Illmatic*, and, like Tony Montana in *Scarface*, no matter what life throws at you, remain valorous on your route to attainment.

Once a target is set, and your inner drive to achieve the aim is at a durable level, your ability to produce in the present becomes the most critical component in the operation, which is why the next chapter is all about flowing in the "now."

Chapter 5

THE ZONE

In 1991, the Chicago Bulls won their first championship in franchise history, defeating the Los Angeles Lakers, four games to one, in a best-of-seven series. Although Los Angeles had stars like Earvin "Magic" Johnson and James Worthy, who have both since been inducted into the prestigious Naismith Memorial Basketball Hall of Fame, the two headliners were no match for the hungry and ever-so-determined Michael-Jordan-led Bulls. In the five games, Jordan averaged a series-high 31.2 points per game, and a team-high 11.4 assists per contest. Because of his otherworldly performances in the set of bouts, Jordan was named the NBA Finals Most Valuable Player (MVP).

Shortly following the series-clinching victory, one of the more iconic photos in NBA history was snapped by photographer Andrew Bernstein, who, with one still shot, captured an incredible moment that showcased Jordan, crying tears of joy while lovingly hugging the championship trophy, with his father clutching his right arm in support of his superstar son. Jordan, who, at that point, had been in the league for seven years, was finally able to reach his goal of winning a title. By gazing at the emblematic snapshot, one can vividly sense the onerous work that Jordan had put in to reach the golden destination.

The very next year, M.J. and the Bulls were looking to run it back and retain their crown as the best team in the land. In the regular season, the Bulls won sixty-seven games, which, at the time, was the most in franchise history. Jordan, for the second year in a row, was named the regular season MVP.

With their eyes on the prize, the top-seeded Bulls marched right into the 1992 playoffs with two emphatic wins over the eight-seed Miami Heat in the first round. Back then, the opening round was best-of-five, so Chicago stood just one victory shy of advancing. However, in Game Three, Miami refused to back down to the defending champions and came out of the gates with vengeance. Within the first ten minutes of the contest, the Heat took an unforeseen eighteen-point lead over the mighty Bulls. What was even more remarkable was the fact that Jordan, who had averaged 39.5 points in the two previous matches, had a whopping zero points.

Basking in this rare, unanticipated moment, Heat fans confidently cheered on their team, as it looked like the underdogs would extend the series and force a Game Four. A victory here would also be Miami's first in franchise history against the Bulls, who had defeated them in all previous sixteen matches dating back to 1988.

Unfortunately for the Heat and their large crowd of passionate supporters, all fifteen-thousand-plus individuals in attendance at the Miami Arena on April 29, 1992, were about to experience history in real time. I used the word "unfortunately" because, right after the Heat's sizzling start, Jordan went bananas and metaphorically silenced the entire city of Miami. In superhero fashion, over the remainder of the tilt, Jordan scored a monstrous fifty-six points to lead the Bulls to a comeback, series-seizing victory, 119–114. At the time, fifty-six points was tied for the third most for a single game in playoff history. The record in this department is sixty-three, held of course by Michael Jeffrey Jordan himself, who accomplished this feat, years earlier, in 1986, against the Larry-Bird-led Boston Celtics.

After the game, when asked about Jordan's prodigious performance, Miami's Rony Seikaly said, "He's like a grenade without the pin." When the media members made their way over to Jordan to capture his immediate thoughts on his historic game, "His Airness" kept his comments short and simple: "I was in *the zone*," said Mike. "I just see myself and the basket. It's a great zone to be in."

"The zone," in positive psychology, is the mental state in which a person partaking in a particular action is entirely imbued with a strong sense of focus, involvement, and amusement. Simply put, it's when you are truly locked-in on whatever you're putting energy toward. It's an upgrade from your normal state, because, in ordinary times, you are in command of what you're thinking about and how you presently feel, whereas being in the zone is a frame of mind where internal dialogue is temporarily silenced and your being synthesizes with the warmth of the moment.

For some, being "in the zone" is a way to classify an individual who appears to be completely present. Those who sustain a lively "flow state," as it's often called, experience a vivid sense of clarity, allowing them to essentially slow down time and perfectly perform en route to easily reaching their desired result in the specific act. This frame of mind can be perceived for those who participate in rather difficult and highly captivating endeavors. In Jordan's case, while competing against some of the top basketball players in the world, M.J. was able to block out not just thousands of screaming fans, but also the opposition, which allowed him to get buckets at will.

While most of us don't know what it's like to have supernatural basketball skills and, time after time, put on uncanny spectacles that routinely have millions in complete awe, there's a good chance that each one of us, at one point or another, has been in a state of mind in which our awareness was heightened, and, because of this, we possessed unwavering focus on the task at hand.

What's appealing about "the zone," as it relates to the human experience, is that complete immersion in an act that one is passionate about almost always results in a strong feeling of elation. When one laughs, they are technically existing in the flow state, as they are entirely operating in the present moment while expressing mirth. If you stop and think about your happiest moments in life, chances are, the majority (if not all) of the mental scenes that you recall are times in which you were in "the zone." Free of thought, and as present as can be. This is why it feels like time flies by when you are with someone you love, because the level of engagement is so deep and profound, to the point where you are fully absorbed in the instant, and lose track of everything external.

Being in "the zone" while operating in your personal craft will give you the best chance for success in the present endeavor, as all extrinsic feelings are nonexistent and the only perceived marker is your desired result. If you've ever put a decent amount of energy toward an appealing area that calls for human expression (writing, drawing, speaking, acting, dancing, singing, athletics, etc.), then you have surely sensed the difference between being somewhat engaged in the activity and being completely locked-in on the pursuit. When you are experiencing the latter, you are like Jordan: immune to any outside noise and able to attack your aim with ease. In extreme cases, being one with the present can feel like an out-of-body episode, as your degree of awareness causes you to perceive the moment from beyond your physical being and observe "the now" through an incredibly deep lens. Hence why Jordan mentioned that, while dominating on the court, it felt

like it was just him and the hoop. Even though there was clearly
a set of competitors whose collective plan was to stop him from
scoring, these players were unsuccessful because they were up
against a being who was in a supernatural headspace.

Awake to this realization, it is apparent that if one wishes to
live life to the fullest and ensure that they come across as many
gratifying and miraculous moments as possible, an evident aim to
set would be to try and consistently interface with reality in a state
of intense clarity. To begin acting toward this intent, one must
first understand what type of experiences allow them to enter the
flow state. Based on the above paragraphs, it is clear that the one
constant for someone to exist in "the zone" is that the being must
possess a deep adoration for whatever, and whoever, they are
putting stamina toward.

In the odd case in which a strong interest is not present for the
actual act, one could also enter "the zone" whenever a clear target
is intensely set that coincides with the performance. When one
possesses a burning desire to materialize a distinct outcome, they
are natively geared to enhance their level of focus throughout
their pursuit to realization.

An example of this would be when you took an important test
in school, one in which the result of the examination weighed
heavily on your overall grade. The actual acts of studying and,
come test time, physically answering the questions probably

weren't that glamorous, but, because of the hefty circumstances, your hunger to succeed in the feat most likely forced you to lock-in on the process. Outside of the classroom, certain individuals who aim to build their own business also experience moments in which they are flowing in the now, especially in the early years, as their need to excel and create wealth is so extreme that they are willing to push through the tedious work and potential hardships in order to reach their lofty goal of creating a blooming operation. A good majority of, if not all, influential pursuits require a lot of energy expended on monotonous and unappealing tasks. Those who flourish in life are those who are so deeply devoted to the destination that they make it a priority to zone in on the repetitive, laborious, and sometimes unpleasant actions in order to accurately actualize their aims.

Putting school and business aside, by planting any supreme intention in your personal passage, you give yourself the chance to perceive life at a crystalline level. This is why the last section was solely centered around setting targets to attack. Not just basic goals, but ones that are meaningful to you and/or challenging to reach. The loftier the objective, the harder one will internally push and zero in on the moment in order to progress toward the finish line. If the bar is not set to the stars, there's no reason to focus on getting to the clouds.

All in all, to exist in "the zone" is to live present, with intense clarity. The three most common ways to naturally enter this headspace are:

1. Loving the activity that you are partaking in.
2. Spending time around people that you deeply appreciate.
3. Establishing purposeful and ambitious marks to propel your internal drive while on the chase for greatness.

For the purposes of this section in the project, I will be exclusively focusing on the importance of being in "the zone" as it pertains to personal attainment. Understanding that a strong blend of devotion and desire helps you perceive life from a luminous lens, which, in turn, aids you in your present pursuit, it is vital to ensure that you familiarize yourself with operating in "the zone," so that when it comes time to lock in at any moment, you are well-acquainted with the elevated experience.

This is where the fitness connection comes into play. As we know, partaking in a fiery physical workout will naturally lead to an enhancement in attentiveness and overall focus, which are two preeminent attributes that are obtained and running while someone is in a flow state. What's interesting about the actual act of exercising is that, when performed correctly, a functioning fellow will inherently dwell in the zone throughout any standard workout.

Let's use the idea of lifting weights, from a general perspective, as an example. Prior to performing the activity, the active individual inherently decides how many pounds are suitable for them to lift with the hopes of successfully completing their desired amount of reps. Let's say a fitness enthusiast aims to do three strong sets of ten bicep curls, and opts to utilize a pair of forty-pound dumbbells to complete the drill. In order to flourish, the being must magnify their internal focus by making sure their muscles are properly extended and retracted, while also controlling their breath and posture. This in-house checklist forces the person to live in the present moment if they wish to propitiously perform.

In the midst of the action, blood from the being's liver and digestive system gets redirected to their skeletal muscles. Fat in their body is converted to glucose, which creates an enhancement in present mood and overall emotional state. As the individual moves through the exercise, lactic acid is produced by the muscles, and, as the contents of it expand, the pH levels of the blood encompassing the muscles decreases. This reduction is what inhibits the muscles from further contracting, which forces the soul to rest and regroup before the next set. While all of this is happening, the brain manufactures the previously referenced neurotransmitters, like dopamine, norepinephrine, and serotonin, and the heart beats faster, which, in turn, enhances blood flow. Increased blood circulation throughout the body is highly beneficial, as it aids in effectively boosting cell growth and organ function. Norepinephrine, which is actually made from dopamine, directly enhances reaction time and overall alertness, helps focus one's attention on the immediate, strengthens one's ability to form and retrieve memories, and aids in regulating blood flow to the skeletal muscles, among many other benefits.

Strong blood circulation spawned from physical exercise comforts the mind and directly elevates one's ability to focus in the moment. A serene mind is well-armed to take on any type of stress-related situation, while a bothered mindset is detrimental for anyone involved in a tension-filled experience. This is why people with high levels of stress will see spikes in their blood pressure, which causes them to have poor circulation. Just by lifting weights, one is able to nest in a flow state and naturally arrange their body to be assembled for success.

Of course, identical benefits are reaped through an aerobic—and truthfully, any intensified physical drill, as well. When someone is in the middle of a run, their heart is profoundly pumping and effectively shifting oxygenated blood to the muscles and brain. Simultaneously, the body discharges endorphins, which triggers the aforementioned "runner's high," which is genuinely another denomination for being in "the zone." When a dedicated sprinter experiences this temporarily enchanted feeling, their brain signals the adrenal glands to generate epinephrine, or "adrenaline," which gives them an energy boost and allows for even more oxygen to get to the muscles.

Fierce exercise, in general, increases the levels of endocannabinoids in the bloodstream. For those unfamiliar, endocannabinoids are lipid-based neurotransmitters, which, when pushed into the brain, provide temporary consciousness-expanding effects like reduced angst and feelings of tranquility. With that said, the release of these mood-enhancing neuromodulators helps put an active individual in a transitorily elevated space.

What's beautiful about "the zone," as it pertains to working out, is that entering this hallowed mental slot is completely effortless. To get there, all you have to do is immerse yourself in the physical activity and, naturally, your state of mind is upraised. The more you exercise, the more you'll instinctively find yourself dispassionately observing the world, absent from thought, and, at times, metaphorically outside of your body. For those who are reading this book as experienced fitness beings, I'm sure you are well aware of what this lifted headspace is like, and, for the individuals that are new to the exercise game, get ready to enjoy life from a profound lens.

As you consume this concept, when it comes to your typical exercise environment, be mindful of the fact that it is easiest to arrive at your mental zenith when working out alone. This is because, in companionless settings, all individuals are innately forced to focus on the task at hand. When you exercise by yourself, you erase any chance of external distraction, thus raising your odds of feeling personally satisfied. Once you've hit a groove in your isolated, physical session, your state of mind will naturally elevate. This is rather meaningful because this high-minded space not only enhances your concentration, but it also allows you to joyfully feel the present, which as we know, is a gift in its own right. As touched on in a past chapter, your level of self-love has a direct impact on the degree to which you're able to appreciate your surroundings. Solo fitness affairs allow you to productively practice your ability to enter "the zone," but, additionally, because of the emotional boost, each workout can also be viewed as a self-appreciation exercise. The more unaccompanied workouts you partake in, the more time you'll spend perceiving the world with a deep devotion for self, which is a win-win-win when it comes to your happiness status, future personal output, and level of positive influence on others. Moreover, enjoying some alone time by way of physical movement is a great way to strengthen your inner warrior. In life, at one point or another, we are all tested by being put into various situations that call for individual persistence—distinct circumstances in which the only soul who can push us forward to the light at the end of the tunnel is the one we see in the mirror whenever we gaze deeply into our personal pair of globular organs. To increase the odds of success in these isolated conditions, we must be able to live happily and effectively in solitary, and the best way to boost our solider spirit is by pushing our physical body while temporarily detached from society. This way, our mind is able to seamlessly slide into a sublime state, and our fleshly frame is urged to go

beyond our standard level of comfort while we put energy toward
the fitness drills. Every time this combination is activated, we
are symbolically bolstering the fighter in all of us. Our inherent
combatant that we will call on in times of battle. A gladiator who
is brave, tenacious, and built for war.

Along with the actual act of exercising, if you're looking for a
boost to skyrocket into the flow state during a workout, listen
to your favorite songs while you perform. As many know, it's
incredibly common for people to jam out to their beloved tunes
while they train, but what's great about the pairing is that past
research has revealed that listening to music in the midst of a
peppy workout can enhance endurance levels, elevate mood,
reduce blood pressure, improve mental alertness, and distract
the mind from any potential feelings of slight pain or tiredness
that the body may be experiencing as a result of the vigorous
exercise. Music has massive effects on both our mental and
emotional states, and when mingled with fitness, it is sincerely
a performance enhancer. There is more research that needs to
be done around the overall influence of melodic sounds, and,
collectively, because of the potentially massive, reality-shifting
findings, we as lively beings should be putting more thought
toward the power of frequencies. Just my two cents.

Anyway, from the big picture, virtually all high-performers have
a strong ability to engross themselves in their desired field, which
gives them the advantage over those who casually compete in

their craft. Those who excel in life are those who have been able to exclusively distance themselves from the pack, and the most efficient way to go about achieving this is by intensely focusing on your area more than everyone else. The late, great Kobe Bryant, a basketball icon who won five championships with the Los Angeles Lakers during his storied twenty-year NBA career, openly outlined the overwhelming value behind this idea to perfection in a 2016 interview that took place on the 126th floor of the Shanghai Tower for a TEDx Salon talk. In the discussion, Bryant, sporting a "FOREVER MAMBA, FOREVER LEGEND" black T-shirt, made note of his fierce training habits and mentioned how habitually waking up early to work out gave him a clear edge over his opponents.

To be the best basketball player you can be, "you have to practice, you have to train," said Bryant, on stage, speaking to a crowd of about sixty lucky listeners at the second tallest building in the world. "You wanna train as much as you can, as often as you can. So if you get up at ten in the morning, train at noon. Train for two hours, twelve to two, you have to let your body recover. You get back out, you train. You start training at six, train from six to eight and now you go home, you shower, you eat dinner, you go to bed, you wake up and you do it again. Those are two sessions."

Without hesitation, and with little to no emotion, Bryant continued. "Now imagine, you wake up at three and you train at four, go four to six, come home, breakfast, relax. Now you're back at it again, nine to eleven, you relax and now, all of a sudden, you're back at it again, two to four. Now you're back at it again, seven to nine. Look how much more training I have done by simply starting at four. So now you do that, as the years go on, the separation that you have with your competitors and your peers just grows larger and larger and larger and larger and larger. By year five or six, it doesn't matter what kind of work they're doing in the summer, they're never gonna catch up."

Kobe Bryant wasn't a great athlete just because he consistently showed up to practice. He was otherworldly because, in the midst of every training session, he was determined to become the greatest basketball player he could possibly be, and that level of unwavering focus, sprinkled with relentless commitment, is what it takes to become the greatest version of yourself.

By regularly exercising, without even realizing it, you are formally training your mind to energetically engage in "the now," so that when it's time for you to heighten your focus in your particular profession, you'll be able to lavishly lock in. The more fitness sessions you tackle, the more acquainted you will become with fixating on any objective. Beyond the physical and intellectual perks, exercising truly teaches you how to be present and mentally raises your level of alertness so that you're steadily in a solid position to effectively spotlight your goals and aspirations.

The purpose of adopting an exercise routine stretches far beyond just appearance and health, which is why it is so important to spread this information in a clear, concise manner, so that you, the reader, are fully awake to the underrepresented rewards. As previously mentioned, at our core, we all want to be happy and successful. By successful, we mean achieving whatever it is that we set out for, and by habitually residing in "the zone" while we exercise, our minds will naturally gravitate toward this elevated state for whenever we signal that it is time to focus and achieve an aim. Life is a race against time, and if you're frequently unable to mentally lock in on the work that requires your undivided attention, moments will pass you by with no remorse, and you will never live out your true potential. This is why it is so critical to spend as much time in the zone as humanly possible. Perceiving life in the present allows us to make the best decisions for the betterment of our personal journey. Although the lead-up to memorable instances in life calls for hours of work, focus, and discipline, in the actual moments of satisfaction, the mind is free of thought, and operating subconsciously. If your mind has not been seasoned to function in "the now," you put yourself at risk for failure when opportunities with small margins for error arise.

Whether you're in the thick of creating a compelling product or service, or constantly operating in any fashion in which your performance levels dictate your overall success, sustaining enhanced perceptivity in your space will undoubtedly put you in the strongest position for victory. Imagine you're taking an eye test, and, as part of the procedure, you are forced to accurately identify and shout out columns of letters that, as you move down the chart, get smaller and smaller in font size. In the first attempt, you do it with two wide-open, healthy eyes, and ace the exam. The second time around, however, you are asked to scrunch up your eyes while analyzing a completely different set of letters, and, unfortunately, you incorrectly classify the symbols because you were squinting. In the final attempt, you are required to close your eyes and run through the assessment with a fresh new set of signs. Of course, you fail miserably, as your one sense needed to prevail was temporarily disabled for the exercise.

These three experiments metaphorically represent what it's like in life to have full mental clarity vs. partial visibility vs. no lucidity at all when attacking any pertinent endeavor. In order to ensure that you're constantly progressing with complete clarity in your craft, you must exist in "the now," and, because of the physical happenings and sensible boosts that take place within your body during a workout, exercising is, by nature, an incredibly powerful activity to safeguard your focus.

If you've been around the block enough times, then chances are you've endured a handful of events in life that regrettably didn't go your way. Ones that you would do anything for another swing at. When you stop and think about any of these unfortunate moments along your journey, you can probably point to a lack of focus as being a predominant cause for the poor result. Many times, without even knowing it, we, as humans, fail to even recognize when we aren't concentrating to our fullest potential. Whether it be too many outside distractions that muddy our vision, or poor influences in our path, the people that fail to capitalize on their opportunities, and always point out that "you don't know what you've got until it's gone," are the souls that lacked present focus when it was needed the most. Knowing the undeniable importance of maintaining a grip on "the now," exercising, for just the boosts in mental clarity alone, should make it a required task for anyone who wishes to sustain success. If there's an activity that will help you concentrate in your day-to-day life, one that will conclusively aid you in your path to achieving your aims, then you must add it to your regimen. It's as simple as that.

Another thought to consider before moving onwards to the next section is the obvious, yet oddly overlooked, value in focusing on things you love. The notion of primarily putting energy toward activities that you adore appears evident, but, for any odd reason, some of us, at times, find ourselves operating in areas that we aren't truly fond of. When we concentrate on what we genuinely appreciate, our whole body blissfully senses the internal desire and dazzling devotion, whereas if we get caught up in scenes that don't appeal to us, the body, depending on how extreme the dislike for the particular endeavor might be, could activate an adverse reaction across multiple areas in our being.

Up to this point in the story, we are already well aware of the lusty effect that love has on the psyche. As a fresh reminder, when we zero in on what, or who, we cherish, our brain passionately produces a healthy dose of neurotransmitters that provide positive perks that allow us to deeply appreciate, and significantly sense, whatever it is that we admire. When a strong level of reverence is present, our state of mind is naturally circuited to profoundly connect with, and concentrate on, the area with which one is infatuated, which allows us to perceive reality from the elevated frame. Comprehending this, it is clear that aiming attention at what you treasure will instinctively put you in an elated mindset, one that has the potential to feel transcendental. This supernatural space cannot be reached if there is a shortage of attachment or desire, so, according to science, if you do not focus on what you love, you'll never exist in your supreme form. This is directly due to the fact that your brain will miss out on the production of the key neurotransmitters, which, as we know, are principally responsible for unlocking your ingrained superpowers. By interacting with reality without fixating on what you prize, you are brazenly suspending the production of miraculous molecules, which is strikingly damaging to your potential output in life.

Grasping the fact that a superb burst of horsepower is generated whenever you zoom in on what you're keen on, it is imperative that you follow your inner nature and use your senses as a personal tour guide for life. How you feel about whatever it is that you're putting energy into will candidly dictate the number of mental enhancements that form in your mind, so operating from within is essential for sweeping success. To come full circle, the more you work out, the deeper you'll be able to sense the feelings of love and happiness, and the better you'll be at existing in the present. This forcible fusion readily helps unveil your highest frame.

Looping in the process of tying your shoes, the more focused you are on your aim, the easier it becomes to achieve the desired result. Within this section, we found that exercising coercively strengthens our ability to zone in on "the now." In life, our objectives can range from elementary to complicated, and the more difficult the desire, the more we need to concentrate on the present moment to ensure that each step is calculated carefully. With a rudimentary act like tying your shoes, based on presumed experience, your level of attention as you operate in the action will most likely not modify your ability to succeed in the feat, yet the basic undertaking will be easiest to achieve if all of your energy is zeroed in on your performance. With harder objectives, in order to increase your reward rate, you need to deliberately block out everything external that could possibly trigger any of your inherent senses. It is believed that the human brain is able to process eleven million bits of information per second, but our conscious minds pick up on no more than sixty bits per second. What this tells us is that our brain does a great job of eliminating more than 99.9 percent of potential input and deems it irrelevant for the moment, yet, because of this, we are limited to what we can handle in "the now." With that said, knowing that there is a limited number of details that your mind can manage per second, it is ever so important that, prior to putting energy toward something of importance, that you obliterate all extrinsic happenings that are not in line with achieving the desired result. Quite obviously, whenever any of your senses are provoked, whether it be sight, smell, taste, hearing, touch, vestibular, or proprioceptive, your brain will immediately steer your attention toward the specific activation. Comprehending this, to get the best results in an action that matters greatly, you must be able to retain explicit control over the finite amount of conceivable information that absorbs your brain's attention each second. Possessing the discipline to consistently command the direction of your attention will do wonders for your existence.

On top of targets varying in complexity, the opportunities in this game that offer you a chance to achieve greatness are limited. Not only are you given a finite number of attempts in life, but, depending on the specific goal, you might only have one shot, and/or a confined window of time, to succeed. Think about a basketball player who gets passed the ball with his/her team down by one point with a few seconds left on the clock. Or a hungry entrepreneur given just three minutes to present his/her product to potential investors. In both situations, the margin for error is so slim that any falter in focus could result in failure. Because of the fixed factors in the two circumstances, the two beings won't have any time to think, and will naturally act subconsciously. Your mind must be able to effectively operate while it's in its subconscious state, and the best way to program it for success is by habitually fixating your attention on the hunted result and everything that comes along with it.

As far as the recipe for success is concerned, this chapter is primarily associated with the third rule. Our level of focus per action heavily influences the amount of time it takes to obtain any objective. Beyond just getting reps in your favored field, with the hopes of getting closer toward achievement, you must constantly measure your internal concentration status for whenever energy is put toward the particular space. Your life is a set of separate stages, and within each level, you only have so much time and stamina to expend in order to create the best results. With that being said, you must be efficient with how you spend your waking hours, and the only way to do so is by being locked in on the present, and entirely fixated on the current mission.

Since our level of concentration on the task at hand plays such a meaningful role in the outcome of the effort, it is essential that we have a clear understanding of how to effectively control our attention. Beyond the subject matter in this section, one of the main factors that determines how well we remain present is our ability to properly breathe. Breathing is a skill, and one that, as a result of recent findings, is becoming increasingly more necessary to master if you wish to live as your strongest self. Fortuitously for active souls, our ability to move air, both into and out of the lungs, is efficaciously enriched each time we put our bodies through an intense exercise.

Chapter 6

BREATHE

All living beings are breathing, but some living beings breathe more efficiently than others. Since it's an involuntary action, most individuals don't take the time, or energy, to polish their inhaling and exhaling technique. Despite how primitive the actual act may appear, each time you gasp for air, there is more going on internally than you could ever imagine, and your performance in the effort can strongly influence your stress levels, blood pressure, feelings of well-being, and overall ability to forcefully function.

The dynamics of a complete breath affect the entire body. On average, humans breathe in and out about 22,000 times per day. Breathing is what keeps the symbolic battery in our beings activated. The explanation of the process is rather elementary: Our lungs service us with oxygen. When we breathe in air, the lungs allow the oxygen to pass into our bloodstream. From there, it is lugged off to the tissues and organs, which allows us to function as lively beings. When we breathe out, our lungs take carbon dioxide from our blood and discharge it into the atmosphere. The better we can breathe, the more we can achieve.

Typically, our lungs become fully developed between twenty and twenty-five years old. Once you hit your mid-thirties, it is common for your lungs to slowly decline in overall performance as the years go by. This is why it's ever-so-important to consistently monitor their capabilities, so that as you age, your breathing remains at the top of its game, and you can continue to operate as a flourishing being.

In order to regularly examine the performance of the pair of organs in your chest that equip your body with oxygen, it would be beneficial to have some background knowledge. Your brain determines the speed at which your lungs are able to gather air. For example, if you're on a run and moving at a brisk pace, your brain will signal to the lungs that they must operate at a quicker rate in order to effectively draw in the invisible gaseous substance surrounding the Earth. On the flip side, when your body is dormant, your lungs are instructed to slow down.

Humans are equipped with two lungs. The left lung has a pair of lobes, while the right lung has a set of three. As far as size goes, the lung on the left side of the body is actually a tad smaller than its counterpart, as space in that area is specifically fitted for the heart. The amount of air that a set of lungs can hold differs from being to being.

Physiological factors that can impact the volume of our lungs include age, gender, weight, height, ethnicity, attitude, and *physical activity*, among others. Taller people have larger lungs, and males, for the most part, have bigger lungs than females. Individuals who habitually exercise have a large lung capacity, which allows them to move oxygen around their body faster than those who don't typically test their cardiovascular system by way of a physical workout. Not only is your body moving the odorless reactive gas at a rapid rate when you exercise, it's also using more of it, which enhances the strength and functionality of your lungs and muscles. Simply put, having a large lung capacity allows the body to efficiently transfer oxygen into the bloodstream and productively ship it over to the active muscles. As many apprehend, having a strong internal system is an indispensable precursor for external eminence.

During a workout, if you're looking to specifically strengthen your diaphragm and the muscles betwixt your ribs that effectively collaborate to propel how you inhale and exhale, both aerobic exercises and any muscle-sharpening drills will be of great benefit. As many know, going for a run, riding a bike, swimming in a body of water, or jumping rope are all great activities for both your heart and lungs, and any type of weight-lifting practice, because of the physical exigencies within the task, will also innately bolster your breathing muscles.

Since this project is focused on the mind-body connection, the goal of this chapter is to disclose how certain breathing procedures impact the brain, and concisely explain what you can do while you exercise to ensure that you are inhaling and exhaling air to your greatest ability. Breathing, as a subject matter, is wildly vast, which makes it hard to conclusively comprehend how exactly we should try to perform the act in order to get the best results. Depending on what you read, particular techniques may appear better than others, but my focus for this project is to simply illustrate what you can do in real time during a workout that, through research, has been shown to positively impact the mind.

Aside from the fact that you're naturally enhancing circulation and toughening the tissue around your lungs amidst a vigorous workout, to truthfully get the most out of an arranged fitness session, you must zone in on your breathing patterns. This is easiest to achieve while working out independently, as the fewer outside distractions, the better, especially as it pertains to enhancing your inner concentration. I consider a deep focus on breathing habits "a must" during a workout because, the more time you spend fixating on your inhaling and exhaling styles, the more natural it will feel to focus on your breathing if, for whatever reason, your attention happens to waver in your everyday life. Dependng on how busy your day-to-day schedule is while on the road to greatness, it could be difficult for some to routinely set aside time and practice effective breathing, so making it a focus point while training allows you to productively knock out two birds with one stone. Plus, concentrating on breathing immediately makes a being more present, and the more locked-in

one is on the moment, the more effective they become. So zeroing
in on the pace and caliber of each breath during a training session
is key if you wish to get the best results.

Without going into too much detail, one way to expertly elevate
your breathing skills in the middle of a workout is to breathe in
consistent clips. Paced breathing, as it's formally called, is when
a human makes a concerted effort to inhale and exhale to a fixed
tempo. For example, let's say you wrap up a set of a particular
drill and you take about forty-five seconds to briefly rest and
let your body recover before launching into the next exercise in
your routine. Instead of erratically breathing to recharge your
body, set some parameters, and track not just the number of
times you gasp and emit air, but also the length of each breath.
This could mean inhaling for a count of three to five seconds, and
exhaling for a count of five to seven seconds. Whatever figures
you select, repeat the process for your elected number of times
before reengaging in the workout. Past research has found that
paced breathing can improve focus and regulate the nervous
system. This, of course, makes sense, as the more zoned in you are
on your breathing habits, the more alert you are, and by adding
numbers to the equation, you trigger certain neural networks
beyond the brain stem that are linked with attention, feeling, and
overall perception.

If you're interested in how exactly this type of focused breathing
relates to our awareness and senses, researchers at the Feinstein

Institute for Medical Research have you covered. For investigative purposes regarding this very topic, a set of experimenters within the research arm of Northwell Health analyzed six adults who were presently in the middle of intracranial EEG monitoring for epilepsy. For those unfamiliar, an EEG is a recording of brain activity, one in which tiny sensors are anchored to a subject's scalp, which allows a medical observer to effectively track the electrical signals that are manufactured by the patient's brain. For the analysis, the participants were petitioned to partake in three unique breathing exercises. For the first drill, the field was told to sit calmly and relax with their eyes open for eight minutes and breathe as they regularly would. Immediately following the eight-minute exercise, the contestants, for about two more minutes, boosted their breathing pace, and for this portion, solely inhaled and exhaled through their noses. This series was repeated eight times.

In the second exercise, the participants were tabbed with keeping track, for two-minute intervals, of how many times they inhaled and exhaled. Once they reported their numbers to the research team, the investigators, who were tightly measuring the breath count of each participant during the drill, jotted down whether the members of the study were accurate or not in their personal claims.

The final practice was an attention-focused drill. Each of the six participants wore a device that recorded their breathing patterns.

As part of the exercise, the contestants looked at a video screen that contained black circles in scattered, but settled, locations. Eventually, the black circles would change color to white, and, as soon as they noticed the switch in hue, the participants were told to press one of four keyboard keys.

Following the evaluation of the trio of exercises, the research team, who firmly examined each participant's rate of breath directly in relation to the specific assignment at hand, conclusively determined that breathing influences the cortex and midbrain much more than experimenters had previously thought. While analyzing the data, the researchers discovered that whenever a participant breathed at an accelerated rate, there would be an increase in activity across a circuitry of brain structures, including the amygdala, which is related to emotion, and specifically plays a key role in how we respond to stressful situations. The uptick in action whenever a participant breathed rapidly allows us to better understand why we tend to inhale and exhale at a speedy rate in nerve-racking moments.

Beyond the emotional element, the researchers also found that when a participant deliberately breathed in a specific rhythm, there was motion in the insula, which is often associated with body awareness and helps manage the autonomic nervous system. Any type of disturbance in this part of the nervous system can affect any body part or process, so it is encouraging to see that a form of measured breathing can help keep a being in line. For those wondering what the data looked like when the contestants correctly announced their breath count in the second exercise, both the insula and anterior cingulate cortex were active, which makes sense. To be accurate in any event, one must obviously possess a certain level of awareness, but it's still reassuring to see certain theories defended by science. All in all, this study is influential because it allows us to confidently state that one's level of focus and present emotional state can be meticulously modified by way of a precise breathing cycle.

If you've ever researched how to dexterously breathe during a specific physical activity, depending on the source, you'll most likely get a handful of different answers. Some experts will recommend that, when running, you'll want to use a distinct two-to-one pattern, which means inhaling twice through the nose, and exhaling once through the mouth. This combination helps to further energize your diaphragm and allows the body to maximize its oxygen intake. Other subject-matter gurus might say to exclusively breathe through the nose during a sprinting session, since nasal breathing, because of the release of nitric oxide in the act, can help you get more oxygen to your tissues than mouth breathing, which does not effectually discharge nitric oxide. In addition, nose breathing is seen as a stronger option than mouth breathing because it helps sift out any foreign particles that you could be exposed to, enhances air flow to arteries, veins, and nerves, monitors the temperature of your breath, humidifies and moisturizes the air, and aids in alleviating any feelings of tension or tightness, among others.

Additionally, from a mental standpoint, primarily breathing through the nose helps elevate one's ability to consolidate their memories, as the actual act vitalizes nerves in the olfactory bulb, which is a rounded mass of tissue that is responsible for our sense of smell. This stimulation generates an alert to our hippocampus, which, as we know, is a part of the brain that helps humans process and retrieve their past experiences. This is why, when we take in a scent that we recall sensing from our past, we can immediately put ourselves back in the specific scene that reminded us of the aroma. A certain aura can make you think of a particular person, or really any active experience you've had in reality. Taking action to adroitly augment your memory is important because strengthening your ability to recall prior happenings automatically helps with your personal development, as the more information you have stored from your journey, the easier it becomes to effectively execute in the present. This invigoration of recollection is not possible by inhaling through the mouth, yet mouth breathing during a particularly intense physical drill could feel more comforting, which ultimately will help in real time with completing any arduous exercise.

No matter what, as a rule of thumb, your intent during a workout, as it pertains to inhaling and exhaling, should be to focus on breathing in a rhythm. The more balanced you are with your breath, the easier it is to operate in the moment. Because of the added perks that come with nasal breathing in comparison to inhaling and exhaling through the mouth, certainly try to mainly breathe through your nose, but don't kick yourself if you find yourself gasping through air using the opening in the lower part of your face.

Along with directing attention toward your pace, make an explicit effort to mix in as many deep breaths as possible. There have been scads of studies published that focus on the relationship between breathing and states of mind, and nearly all distinguished sources outline the potential for diaphragmatic breathing—a type of breathing technique in which a being consciously uses their diaphragm to take deep breaths and ultimately utilizes their lungs to the highest ability—to enhance mental performance, stabilize blood pressure, slow the heartbeat, and diminish any negative physiological consequences that might spawn from stressful situations. If you're curious with how this works, in as elementary an explanation as possible, your aforementioned autonomic nervous system is made up of three divisions: the sympathetic nervous system, the parasympathetic nervous system, and the enteric nervous system. The sympathetic nervous system, in particular, manages the body's compulsory response to threatening or stressful situations. When you breathe deeply, meaning you entirely engage your stomach, abdominal muscles, and diaphragm in the act, you're able to effectively stabilize this sector, which in turn slashes feelings of angst and helps place your being in a state of calmness. This is vital to instill during a workout because the physical demands within a toilsome drill create tension on the body, so being able to counteract the uneasiness through a sound breathing tactic is key. Not only will breathing deeply soothe a soul in real time when under physical duress, it will also ameliorate the mind and truthfully train it to remain relaxed whenever a being is placed in a situation in reality that could create physical or mental pressure within. The more times you test your mental strength by routinely putting your body through punishing workouts, the more it'll get used to forcefully functioning in sapping scenes. If you make it a point to breathe deeply during your fitness sessions, your mind will get used to staying in a serene space while strained, and naturally become properly programmed to productively react whenever you find yourself in a nerve-racking situation. It's all just repetition, and the constant fixation on your breathing habits is what's most important when it comes to punctiliously molding the mind.

Briefly speaking on the mental-elevation portion of particular inhale-exhale techniques, for years, the physicians, religious leaders, philosophers, and scholars of Japanese descent have been fascinated with the concept of deep breathing, and all the powers that come with accurately performing the process. Training designed around breath work has been a part Japan's culture since Buddhism and Taoism were first introduced to the country as religious options, which dates all the way back to the fifth century BCE. Tanden breathing, the act of breathing slowly into the lower abdomen, in particular, has been a steadily studied subject for quite some time in the "Land of the Rising Sun," and recent examinations conducted by academics have allowed us to precisely pair science with prior philosophical thoughts centered around the substance.

Just for some background knowledge on the matter, in 1757, Zen Master Hakuin Ekaku (1686–1769), who is widely regarded as one of the most prominent figures in the history of Japanese Zen Buddhism, wrote a book built around Zen teachings titled *Yasen Kanna*, which, in English, translates to "idle talk on a night boat." Throughout his youth, Hakuin habitually studied meditation-based Buddhism in assorted temples across Japan. In the story, Hakuin outlines a period in his life (between ages twenty-six and thirty-one) in which he suffered from "meditation sickness," which, based on his descriptions of the disturbance, sounds like tuberculosis, pleurisy, a nervous breakdown, or some mix of all three. In an attempt to overcome the illness, Hakuin took the healing actions recommended at the time, as he tried medicine, and even underwent acupuncture, but was ultimately unsuccessful in his attempt to effectively regain his health. Looking for better options to get back on his feet, Hakuin travelled to the mountains of Kyoto to pay Hakuyū, a hermit (person who lives alone and is completely separated from society) a visit. Hakuin had heard about Hakuyū, and, aside from his isolation, knew that the man was a master when it came to his

understanding of introspective meditation, and how certain
stillness-based methods can create wondrous outcomes in reality.
Once he arrived, Hakuin explained his ailment in great detail to
the seasoned savant who, upon reflection, provided the feeble
male with a secret technique that required him to close his eyes,
rest in a particular manner, and draw his attention down to the
lower part of his body, so that his energy was felt below the lower
Tanden, and all the way down to the undersurface of his feet.
Once Hakuin successfully instilled the practice, and adopted
further suggested exercises from Hakuyū, over time, he recovered
from the abnormal condition and completely reclaimed his
stamina. Because of this striking physical health rejuvenation,
Hakuin mingled aspects of Hakuyū's teachings into his own
practices and publications. In *Yasen Kanna*, along with preaching
Hakuyū's magical wisdom, Hakuin, while highlighting the
importance of breathing, cited both an old Korean physician and
a Chinese philosopher. The quotations, translated, read: "The true
person breathes from his heels while the ordinary person breathes
from his throat," and "When the vital energy is in the lower heater
(lower Tanden), the breaths are long; when the vital energy is in
the upper heater, the breaths are short."

In 2004, Masaki Fumoto, Ikuko Sato-Suzuki, Yoshinari Seki,
Yuko Mohri, and Hideho Arita guided a study that further
investigated the spiritualistic, mythical-sounding shifts that
spawn from Tanden breathing, and with modern technology,
the group of scholars came away with some pretty phenomenal

conclusions. In the experiment, the researchers, who analyzed twenty-two healthy participants (aged twenty-one through fifty-four) using an EEG, meticulously inspected the believed-mental effects of Tanden breathing at three to four cycles per minute (inhalation for six to eight seconds, and exhalation for nine to twelve seconds). In the study, electromyography (EMG), which scans electrical activity in response to a nerve's stimulation of a muscle, was recorded to track abdominal muscle contraction, so that the research team was able to confirm whether or not the participants were correctly performing the breathing technique. Of course, if members in the field were to just breathe deeply without anyone analyzing the accuracy in their attempts, there is a good chance that the data would be inaccurate.

As soon as the participants had a firm grip on the fascinating inhale-exhale process, the team began to mark the data. Once the testing phase was complete, the academics reviewed the reports and found that, according to an article about the study published on ResearchPad, "when abdominal breathing (twenty minutes) was performed with eyes closed, low-frequency EEG alpha waves were replaced with high-frequency alpha waves, and subjective vitality increased." Which is a fancy way of saying that the particular breathing procedure promptly raised the participant's frequency levels to a state in which they were immediately able to sense friendly feelings of peace, joy, and love, and were simultaneously given a boost in energy.

In addition, urinary serotonin levels increased significantly after the people took part in the abdominal breathing exercise, which allowed the scholars who spearheaded the study to conclude that "the activity of serotonin neurons in the brain elicited such EEG changes." From here, we can confidently note that, by using our stomach, abs, and diaphragm while breathing, we can actually generate more serotonin in our bodies to create feelings of well-being and truthfully boost our ability to learn and effectively retain past memories. These findings are ever-so-influential because they provide us with clear-cut evidence that scientifically illustrates the potent benefits that an active being reaps from breathing deeply. Yes, it's nice to read about Hakuin's personal path and his scripted beliefs around energy and breath control, but knowing the actual effects that a form of adnominal breathing has on our alpha waves and serotonin status gives us a strong level of assurance, and should emphatically encourage each one of us to habitually concentrate on our breathing habits.

As far as the attention aspect of deep breathing is concerned, in essence, there's a nucleus stationed in the brain stem called the locus coeruleus, where the previously specified neurotransmitter norepinephrine, responsible for enhancing alertness and overall concentration, is created. When you inhale, the activity in this part of the brain stem increases, and when you exhale, it decreases, which tells us that our attention is heavily inspired by our breath. Just by making a purposeful effort to take slow, deep inhales, you are able to fine-tune your focus levels, putting you in a prime position for prosperity in the present.

Something to also keep in mind when thinking about breathing tactics while training is the fact that there are predominately higher levels of oxygen outside in the fresh air than in the air inside. Not only that, but indoor air is two to five times more polluted than outdoor air. This matters greatly because the brain absorbs 20 percent of the oxygen that we inhale, so, based on logic, if you were aiming to take the highest-quality breaths, and suitably service your brain during a workout, the most ideal decision to make would be to exercise outside. More oxygen means more serotonin, and the fresher the air, the better it is for not just your lungs, but ultimately your mood, blood pressure, heart rate, digestive system, and overall energy status. Not to mention the added sun exposure to help raise your vitamin D levels. Obviously, there's nothing wrong with weight-training centers or really any indoor fitness hubs, but it's always important to highlight even the subtlest differences for those who are looking to take the most effective actions possible.

As a whole, the science of breathing is rather sophisticated, and at times, an excessive use of intellectual findings in any area can be somewhat counterproductive, as it can be hard to instill new habits during your waking hours if the information is over-the-top or convoluted. The key takeaways in this section would be to make a premeditated effort to focus on your breath, inhale and exhale in a stable tempo, do your best to primarily breathe through your nose, exercise outside when you can, and make sure you take as many slow, deep breaths as possible. Aside from that, bask in the earlier-voiced benefits for your lungs that add up each time you exercise. While enhancing capacity, and improving how your lungs function as a whole, doesn't sound as alluring as getting stronger muscles and a plethora of mental boosts, these perks for the organs in your chest are not to be overlooked. Your lungs supply your being with oxygen and keep all of the other organs running by clearing carbon dioxide from your body. To continue creating the ideal reality for yourself, you need oxygen, and without well-functioning lungs, you put yourself at serious risk. Even the slightest internal impediment can be inimical to personal growth, so consistently taking the essential actions to avoid inherent issues is pivotal.

Separate from the health-specific portion, a frequent focus on your breathing habits will undoubtedly aid you while on the quest for achievement in all areas of your life. Along with concentrating on how well you're able to inhale and exhale in the midst of an exhilarating exercise, I would highly recommend setting aside time each day to immerse yourself in some type of mindfulness practice. In this reality, the more energy you expend focusing on people you love, hobbies you're fond of, and interests that you're enamored by, the stronger your connection and overall affection levels will be in those personal departments. This rationale is also applicable when it comes to time spent focusing on self. A strong

amount of stamina disbursed toward a self-reflection practice
leads to a healthier bond, and a deeper level of devotion toward
your own character.

If you analyze high-performing individuals in this realm, you'll
find that the lion's share of them habitually isolate themselves
from the world and peacefully sit alone in silence, not only
to sharpen their focus and align with their aims, but also to
harmoniously balance their souls. When one absorbs all of
their attention in a pensive practice, they are able to equitably
energize their being with the symbolic sauce that grants them
the power to effectively exist in an even-keeled manner, which,
in turn, inspires the individual to focus on living a life filled
with love, joy, and prosperity. This is because, in the midst of
a meditative session, once you have completely calmed down
your thoughts, you become the captain of your soul's ship, a title
that allots you the power to steer your emotional state in any
direction you choose. Without even focusing on a clear intention
in thought, if you just concentrate on breathing deeply during a
self-introspective session, you'll inherently garner the emotional
and mental perks that blossom from effectively inhaling and
exhaling in respiration. If your aim is to gain clarity on specific
desires that you wish to see manifested in reality, simply remain
focused on the depth of each breath, and simultaneously, envision
your ideal. While meditating, in the twinkling of an eye, through
clear visualization, your mind and body can sense what it's like
to win a meaningful prize in your chosen craft, even if you're

technically dwelling in a space that contains a dusty, desolate trophy case. You can sense your future wife, who possesses an aromatic aura, and looks stunningly similar to Rachel McAdams, all while individually lying in a practically odorless place. The feeling of observing a set of well-formed waves within a splendid sea on a balmy beach comprised of potently scented sand in the heart of summer can be experienced in a cold setting without a body of water in sight. The pleasurable charm you get when you lovingly listen to your favorite music album with the windows down in your car, excitedly cheer for your cherished sports team after a masterful moment that abruptly changes the course of the competitive outcome, or devotedly watch one of your beloved movies during a scene in which the star of the film injects a healthy dose of inspiration into your spirit, can all be recognized in a room of complete and utter silence. As the commander of your mental state, you're awarded the ability to manage the present status of your mood, which is inarguably one of the more dynamic superpowers that one could ever attain. Through steady self-reflection, you will develop this attribute, and be gifted the strength to productively quarterback your journey in the most satisfying manner possible by harnessing the skill of emotional control. Simultaneously, the more time you invest in abiding in a positive headspace, the more you'll want to call this forward-looking frame of mind your permanent residence, and when that lease is officially signed, you put yourself in a pleasing position to advance in life with ease.

The art of meditating, and genuinely any type of stillness session, is far too extensive to decorously cover in this fitness-based project, but fortunately, there are plenty of pertinent resources across various forms of media to assist anyone who is looking to learn more. Your goals during an introspective sitting should be identical to the breathing targets that you would want to set ahead of each workout: inhale and exhale in a rhythmic pattern, consciously take slow, long breaths, and intentionally suppress any current thoughts that may be running around in your mind so that you can productively place yourself in the present. Even just ten minutes a day solely dedicated to mindfulness has been shown to boost a being's emotional well-being, attention levels, effectiveness in their personal pursuit, and overall health.

No matter what, if you're going to perform a critical action over twenty thousand times per day, you should undoubtedly make it a priority to focus on how well or poorly you're operating in the effort. Obviously, because there's only a finite amount of time to create, and you only have so much stamina to expend, it's nearly impossible to lock in and track the status of every breath, but that's beside the point. What's important is that you fixate on your breathing behavior during your workout, and whenever else you can concentrate on it throughout your day. Knowing that deeply inhaling from the diaphragm is a lot healthier and a much stronger action than slight, upper chest breathing, if you truly aspire to exist in your greatest form, you must persistently aim attention at how exactly you're transporting air in and out of your lungs. If you do not routinely focus on your breathing process, you willfully accept the fact that you're functioning as a fraction of your highest self.

This section's segment on the shoe hypothesis is somewhat of a spitting image to the slice in the last sector. As you take on missions in life that are more comprehensive and drawn-out than lacing up your kicks, your ability to dwell in "the now" will matter more and more. When on the prowl for glory, meaning en route to routinely realizing detailed desires, it is absolutely imperative that you're able to maintain a high level of focus for whenever you dedicate time and energy toward those intentions. The degree to which you have command over your breathing patterns plays a direct role in your capacity to concentrate and exist in the present, which is frankly one of the most important elements to master when it boils down to whether or not you will succeed in a specific act. As we've come to learn, how you customarily breathe impacts your heart rate, emotional grade, energy status, and attention level. Discerning the different results that come with various forms of breathing, in order to thrive in this reality, you need to be able to use your inhales and exhales as savvy tools to help you lock in on the task at-hand. If you watch people perform in truthfully any discipline, ahead of a specific success/failure situation and/or a period in which an entity must aim all of their attention on an act in order to produce an effective outcome, you will see a lot of individuals take a strong, deep breath right before their specific undertaking. Each time the fabled, forenamed

ballplayer Ichiro Suzuki stepped into the batter's box to face
the opposing pitcher, he would take a deep breath, and, while
gripping his bat with his right hand, extend the smooth wooden
club at arm's length toward the pitcher's mound. Simultaneously,
he would tug at his right shoulder sleeve with his left hand. These
actions were adamantly taken for every single at-bat, with the
purpose being to help the hitter adequately align his attention
so that he was in the best position possible to produce a positive
result. While your personal routine for locking in immediately
ahead of an important moment does not need to be as peculiar
as Ichiro's, make sure you incorporate taking a deep breath to
garner the advantages. All professions that are worth pursuing are
highly competitive, and come with such small margins for error,
so even a slightly obscure factor, like leveraging the power of your
breath, can make a massive difference in whether or not you'll be
able to climb.

As far as the recipe for goal-achievement goes, a genuine fixation
on the pace and depth of your breaths will definitely assist
you when it comes to understanding your hunted target, the
confidence you possess in your abilities, and your success rate
when partaking in each act. Setting aside time each day to focus
on your breath will natively place your mind in the present, which
allows you to essentially stop the clock and concentrate on what
your true inner being is trying to communicate to you. At this
point in time, no one really knows where our thoughts originate
from; however, we are able to understand that all information

that hatches in our minds comes paired with a particular emotion that physically alters how we feel. The more pleasing the thought, the better our body reacts to the material. When we sit in silence, temporarily sequestered from reality, and solely focus on our breathing, we are able to attentively tune in to our inner voice and completely sense how our being responds to certain concepts. This practice allows us to identify with particular objectives that we would like to see materialized in reality, and, as we've learned, the clearer the vision, the easier it is to obtain. The more you focus on the dream, from both a mental and a physical standpoint, the more confidence you'll have in the probability of it coming to life.

Again, this chapter was scripted to highlight how your lungs benefit from consistent exercise, and how a focus on your breathing style during a workout plays a part in your overall performance. The additional tidbits around the science of breathing, and mental enhancements that stem from certain mindfulness practices, were provided to inspire you to frequently spotlight the manner in which you inhale and exhale. My hope is that, by continuously advising you to concentrate on your breath while physically working out, you'll not only improve your ability in your drills, but, because of the positive benefits netted while training, you'll be more prone to think about your breaths while actively operating in your day-to-day life.

The idea of consistently concentrating on your breath may feel irrelevant and somewhat minor when it comes to creating your desired results, but trust me, it's not. Blooming beings in this realm excel primarily because they do the little things better than everyone else. They map out their days, which allows them to have a clear understanding of what they will be putting energy toward. They develop self-discipline, and routinely show up even at times when they don't necessarily want to. They follow their heart. They carry an unshakeable belief in their power to shine, and, lastly, they habitually utilize the power in their breath as an energetic engine to drive them as they take on their ambitions.

At this point in the book, we have heavily examined how regularly exercising plays a vital role in an *active* being's ability to succeed. Changing it up a bit, but still staying true to the overarching message, the next section outlines how a person who physically trains benefits greatly during their *inactive* mode.

Chapter 7

SLEEP IS THE COUSIN OF SUCCESS

Getting a good night's sleep tonight will undoubtedly put you in a prime position tomorrow to productively apply your energy in whatever it is that you're chasing. Much like breathing, going unconscious for recharging purposes is something we do so much that we often forget to even think about the quality of our resting sessions. If you average eight hours of sleep per night, you'll spend a third of your entire human existence completely dormant. Knowing this, if you long to live as your greatest self, meaning you strive to effectively maximize your personal output throughout your waking hours, it's important to understand the ins and outs of sleep, and how your snoozing habits coincide with your physical and mental strength.

In the midst of every shuteye session, your brain rotates between REM (rapid-eye movement) sleep and non-REM sleep. As soon as you make an effort to go unconscious, your brain enters the first of four non-REM sleep phases. Since this story is scripted around physical training, let's stay on theme, and illustrate the various sleeping stages symbolically through an aerobic activity. Imagine we are on a regulated running track, and our goal is to run one mile, which, as many know, translates to four loops around the course. For this analogy, each lap represents a different element of non-REM sleep. In the first leg, your body is seesawing between being awake and being knocked out. The next circle around the route symbolizes the period in which your being is softly sleeping. Here, your heart rate and breathing patterns become regulated, and your body temperature begins to decrease.

The final two laps typify deep sleep. Stage three, in particular, has been shown, through recent findings, to influence our ability to learn new information, and retain and recall past memories. In a simple explanation, when you're at your best within this phase of deep sleep, meaning your muscle activity is substantially reduced and your heart rate is at its lowest level, slow waves of electrical activity ride through the brain. These gradual waves allow the brain to productively ship memories from the hippocampus to other areas in the brain that are in charge of permanently storing information. Additionally, because of the fact that your body produces the bulk of its human growth hormone (HGH) for the day during this sleep period, non-REM sleep is vital for the repairing and restoration of your muscles.

About ninety minutes into being unconscious, your body begins REM sleep. This is where the phase's title comes to life, as your eyes, while shut, physically start to shift rapidly from side to side. The waves moving through your brain are nearly identical to those during wakefulness, and your breath rate escalates. Here is where your body becomes transitorily inert as you dream.

Throughout a typical sleeping session, this outlined course continuously repeats itself about four or five times. However, with each succeeding series, you spend less time in the latter half of non-REM sleep, and more time resting in REM sleep.

Much as non-REM sleep influences memory, REM sleep appears to play a part in affecting your critical thinking, creativity, and problem-solving skills. In one specific study designed around this subject, researchers gathered a group of people together and housed them in a sleep laboratory, where the participants had electrodes placed on their heads and, between snoozing sessions, were tested on their ability to accurately solve anagram puzzles (SAVE = VASE, SADDER= DREADS, etc.). Rearranging letters of an established word to create a new word is an easy and ideal way to assess someone's power to think creatively and ultimately solve a puzzle in an able manner, and, by tracking brain activity, the research team was able to accurately analyze how a participant's answer corresponded with their sleeping stage.

For the experiment, the field answered a handful of anagram puzzles and then were asked to doze off. The participants were then woken up four times during the practice to iron out more anagram puzzles. For the purposes of the data, the members in the experiment were awakened twice during non-REM sleep, and twice during REM sleep. After the study was complete, the research team discovered that when the participants were woken up during REM sleep, they were able to solve 15 to 35 percent more anagram puzzles than they could when they attempted the brainteasers after getting woken up in the midst of non-REM sleep.

In a similar study, led by Sara Mednick, PhD, assistant professor of psychiatry at the University of California, San Diego School of Medicine, subjects in the experiment were exposed to a specific set of three words, and then asked to come up with a fourth word that corresponded with the original trio. For example, if the first three words were cookie, heart, and sixteen, an appropriate answer could be "sweet," as cookies are a delectable dessert, a lover is often classified as a "sweetheart," and a common term for a sixteen-year-old's birthday bash is "sweet sixteen." Again, another compelling exercise to determine how various sleep stages may influence the arrangement of associative networks in our most complex organ.

By design, the participants were tested once in the morning, and then once again in the afternoon after they awoke from a nap with either REM sleep, early stage non-REM sleep, or deep-stage non-REM sleep. What's compelling about this study is that the researchers found that the non-REM sleep groups didn't show any signs of improvement on the test over their score from the morning, yet the REM sleep group surpassed their morning scores by nearly 40 percent.

Based on these two studies, it's safe to suspect that REM sleep directly elevates one's adroitness as it appertains to clever problem-solving, and potentially, ingenuity as a whole. So when people advise you to "sleep on it," whenever you are stuck on a particular creative problem and/or need additional time to think about a certain scenario, simply pose the question in your mind, fall into REM sleep, and you might just wake up with a powerful solution. Additional research needs to be conducted on the explicit happenings within the brain during REM sleep to further back the previous analysis up, but there are already plenty of cases in which individuals in this realm credited a dream, or a good night's sleep, as the main reason they were able to solve a unique artistic problem, and/or effectively express themselves in their creative field. An inspiring, textbook example of this would be the origin story behind Train's hit song, "Drops of Jupiter (Tell Me)," which, upon its release in January of 2001, practically skyrocketed the rock band into a supreme sonic-based stratosphere that not many musical acts have reached.

For those unaware of the group's melodic tune, the lyrics, written by lead vocalist Pat Monahan, derive from a spiritual visit paid to Pat by his late mother, who passed away from cancer in December of 1998. Despite the unimaginable loss, Pat, because of the band's strong debut album released that same year, was forced to keep the wheels spinning in order to help his troupe build on the success that they had been grinding for ever since their formation in 1993. By early 1999, Train began to work diligently on their sophomore album, but, after a full year of tirelessly laboring and churning out new material, the crew's music label believed they still needed a smash single to go along with the project.

Still grieving the loss of his mother, and now urged by the record company to promptly produce a sensational track, Pat was in search of answers. However, on one particular night, Pat hit the hay, and, by way of magic, was gifted with a dose of inspiration from his beloved caregiver. In a 2008 interview with VH1's *Behind the Music*, Monahan detailed the occurrence:

"The process of creation wasn't easy," he explained. "I just couldn't figure out what to write, but then I woke up from a dream about a year after my mother passed away with the words 'back in the atmosphere'… It was her way of saying what it was like—she was swimming through the planets and came to me with drops of Jupiter in her hair."

With just a few pieces to the puzzle, Pat, through lucid symbolism, put together the remainder of the pleasurable piece, and, as they say, the rest was history. Following its release, the song won a pair of Grammy Awards, one for Best Rock Song, and another for Best Arrangement, which was written by Paul

Buckmaster. As of 2022, the hit song has over 600 million streams on Spotify alone.

Other massive musical records that allegedly stem from otherworldly visions include Jimi Hendrix's "Purple Haze," The Police's "Every Breath You Take," and The Beatles' "Let It Be." Beyond extracting themes and verses in a rhythmic sense, certain esteemed individuals from our world's history have also endorsed the mere act of falling asleep as an effective way to spark ideas across various endeavors. In particular, surrealist Salvador Dali and inventor Thomas Edison, when in need of some creative inspiration, would both perform a similar, yet incredibly unique, napping method. According to an article in *Smithsonian* magazine, the two influential beings "tried to sleep while holding a small object in their hands, which would then clatter to the floor and wake them up just as they started to doze off. When they woke, they'd go straight to work." Dali, specifically, following a mentally taxing day of ruminating over possible motifs that he wanted to artistically express in his work, would sit in a chair, and softly hold onto a group of keys. Before he would attempt to doze off, the Spanish artist would place a metal tray on the floor and hang the hand that was loosely gripping the keys on the edge of the chair, so that it was directly in line with the plate on the ground. As soon as Dali fell asleep, he would drop the keys and they would smash onto the tray, creating a ringing noise, which would immediately wake him up. This strange sleeping process would give him the creative jolt that he was striving for, and, in similar fashion to the science behind Hakuin's breathing technique, modern research has defended this unconventional resting exercise. In a study led by Delphine Oudiette, a neuroscientist at the Paris Brain Institute, a group of 103 participants were each given a consecutive strand of eight numbers that were specifically spread apart by a particular pattern, and the goal of the assignment was to accurately identify the ninth number that explicitly goes along with the preceding sequence.

In the first go-round, 16 of the 103 members of the field answered the brainteasers correctly. The other 87 were asked to take a twenty-minute rest in which they were connected to a machine that effectively monitored their brain waves. In equivalent fashion to Dali, each individual was required to cradle an object in their hands. If the object were to fall, meaning the entity fell asleep, the being was told to yell aloud their stream of thoughts as they came out of the brief rest.

The field was broken down into three groups: one comprised of those who were able to effectively perform the technique in Dali-fashion, meaning they drifted into an early non-REM stage, but were able to rapidly arise once their object hit the ground; another made up of people who fell into a deeper stage of sleep; and the last one consisting of those who stayed awake during the interval.

From here, they were asked to solve more questions, and the results were quite stunning. A staggering 83 percent of those in the shallow non-REM stage were able to find the pattern that they had failed to pick up on before, and accurately answered the questions. For those who stayed awake, only 30 percent were correct in their pursuits, and amongst the individuals who got a deep, quality rest, a measly 14 percent were able to crack the codes.

Although additional analysis is certainly needed to truthfully make any concrete conclusions, it is safe to assume that there is some sort of sweet spot right between active awareness and sleep that appears to provide a being with an injection of ingenuity and understanding.

While the above information does not directly pertain to physical fitness and its relationship to sleep, it's important to set the stage and lay out recent research and claims from the culture so that you have a clear understanding of, not just the various phases of rest, but also actual actions you can take to put yourself in a position for success. Although this product is built around exercise and the otherworldly benefits that come with consistently working out, if there is previously discovered data related to the theme of the chapter that could potentially help you morph into your greatest form, it must be mentioned.

One of my objectives as the author of this story is to inspire you to soak up this important information and effectually use it in your own path so that you can productively transform into your highest self. A lot of people think of sleep as simply a resting period, but it is clear that going temporarily unconscious has a recognizable effect on our mind and possibly our future reality. Putting aside the timing and specific stage of sleep one was at when they awoke, if you scan these studies at face value, you can safely postulate that dozing off naturally assists us with present hurdles that our attention is actively fixated on. If that's true, which it appears to be, then the thoughts that are racing around our minds immediately before entering an inactive state seem to be incalculably important. The detected data illustrated how a lively being's ability to propitiously perform in an action was distinctly altered after a period of dormancy, which, as a result, modified the human's reality. In each experiment, the sole barrier between whether or not a participant was able to turn his/her negative result into a positive one was a special stretch of sleep. Knowing this, it is essential to be very mindful of the ideas and overall information circulating in your brain right before you knock out. To precisely embrace this analysis and intertwine the findings into your own existence, next time you go to get some rest, consciously think about a certain situation in your life that is either giving you trouble, and/or, through proper execution, is something that you would like to see realized in this realm. Whatever the case may be, right before falling asleep, understand the ideal end result that you aspire to see played out, meticulously ruminate over it, and dwell in the feelings, without resistance, that correspond with crossing the finish line. Assume the objective is fulfilled, as you must possess unwavering faith in your ability to execute in any act, and simply doze off. As we've come to learn, your brain will inherently work toward an effective solution for whatever is attracting your attention and naturally provide you with the knowledge needed to successfully operate in the action.

How this all works is still relatively unclear, but that's not a concern. At this point in time, we are already able to test a human's ability to produce a particular result in an exercise and, through the sleep-related research, declare that briefly going unconscious appears to, in some fashion, readily help uncover the answer to a distinct question that the analyzed being was recently focused on.

Along with learning about the stages of sleep and the pure performance-enhancing techniques that one can put to the test during a resting session, it is also important to accentuate the investigated actions that one can take in order to put themselves in a position for a quality stretch of shuteye. The better you are at sleeping, the better your brain will function during a static period. Of course, a powerfully performing brain makes it easy to garner the mental improvements that naturally spawn from effectively reposing. Here are a handful of organic, professionally cited recommendations to aid an individual in their quest for a stupendous shuteye session:

- No use of electronic devices as you attempt to
  rest (reduce all blue light exposure in evening for
  strongest results).

- Enhance exposure to bright lights (specifically natural
  sunlight) throughout your waking hours.

- Stay consistent with your sleep schedule.

- Avoid caffeine consumption at least eight hours before
  lying down.

- Ensure that the factors in your sleeping space
  (temperature of the room, noise, lighting, mattress/
  pillow quality, etc.) are aligned with your optimal
  resting environment.

- Refrain from eating at least four hours prior to sleep.

- Shy away from liquids at least one or two hours before
  going to bed.

- Take a bath or shower within ninety minutes prior
  to resting.

And, most prominently, exercise regularly. Because of its brisk
ability to operate as a mood stabilizer, and, as a whole, help the
mind unwind, the act of exercising naturally places the brain
in a fantastic position for a first-rate round of rest. Obviously,
from a bodily perspective, a strong amount of physical activity
will inherently generate an eagerness to snooze. Within our
body, all of us have what's called a homeostatic sleep drive,
which is a process that enhances our need to temporarily shelve
consciousness while we are alert. Scientifically explaining how
this works, adenosine, a chemical found in human cells that's

related to our energy status, has three unique forms: adenosine, adenosine monophosphate (AMP), and adenosine triphosphate (ATP). As we exhaust our internal energy throughout the day, ATP is broken down and, as a result, the basal forebrain releases adenosine, which directly increases our desire to sleep. As we rest, it is believed that the buildup of adenosine is cleared from the brain, which allows the being to become revitalized upon activation.

Staying on topic, this mechanism can be symbolically visualized as an air mattress that progressively puffs up during our active hours while we discharge both mental and physical energy. When we go dormant, the metaphorical mattress gradually deflates until we begin our next mobile session. If we were to habitually exercise, our brain would release a lot of adenosine, allowing our emblematic mattress to balloon at a faster pace, which naturally would increase our success rate in regard to the time it would take for us to fall asleep on any given attempt. A group of researchers conducting a study involving older adults who reported moderate sleep complaints actually put this concept to the test and found that consistently exercising cut down the amount of time it took, on average, for a participant to fall asleep by nearly 50 percent. In addition, the field revealed that the moderate-to-intense aerobic drills required in the experiment added forty-one more minutes of sleep per night, which shows how even something as simple as a daily brisk walk can improve quality of rest throughout any given session. If you are one who pushes yourself to the extreme within each workout, meaning you exude a tenacious ton of physical and mental energy, you can expect to naturally increase both the time it takes for you to fall asleep, and the overall caliber of your stretch of stillness.

In another sleep-related study, in which adolescents were the focal point, similar observations to the ones plucked in the case of the sleep-deprived adults were made. After evaluating a group of kids throughout a twelve-week exercise program (180 minutes per week of either an aerobic exercise or some type of resistance training), the researchers guiding the experiment declared that— by way of polysomnography, which is a test that records one's brain waves, oxygen levels, heart rate, and breathing—consistent physical training was shown to decrease the time spent in the first stage of non-REM sleep, and increase REM sleep, sleep continuity, and sleep efficiency.

As far as the timing of your workout goes, the advised slot is still up in the air. There is a lot of research out there, in reference to quality of sleep at night, that illustrates how exercising in the morning is a better option than later in the day. However, you can also find opposing statistics that will swing you in the other direction. No matter what, from an overarching standpoint, the taxing energy exuded from exercising will naturally enhance a being's desire to seek out rest. Physical training does stimulate the aforesaid sympathetic nervous system, so giving your body time for the invigoration in the specified network of nerves to diminish is recommended. All things considered, as long as you don't work out and then, moments later, attempt to fall asleep, you'll be in a strong position for a steady run of rest.

Additionally, the more you exercise, the better control you'll have over the status of your weight, which matters greatly as it relates to sleep. Those who are overweight put themselves at high risk of experiencing symptoms of obstructive sleep apnea (OSA), which barricades a portion, or all, of your upper airway while you're inactive. Suffering from this disorder directly affects the flow of oxygen to your organs and forces your diaphragm and chest muscles to push harder than usual, which, as a result, inhibits your ability to sleep well.

From an anatomic standpoint, there are sundry structures within the brain that are heavily active during a time of rest. Some of these complexes are also heavily influenced while an individual physically exercises. For example, when you temporarily suspend consciousness, your amygdala, the previously referenced almond-shaped structure involved in processing emotions, becomes progressively more and more astir during REM sleep. As we know, by exercising, a being activates the sectors in the brain that are in charge of regulating how effectively we plan, focus our attention, multi-task, and retain information, which, as a result, helps control the amygdala. Running, as a drill by itself, has been shown to provide the amygdala with a positive functional kinship with the orbitofrontal cortex and insula to create a sense of happiness following completion of the cardiovascular-centered activity. Putting two and two together, the more alive and positively operating your amygdala is during the day, the stronger its performance will be at night.

In similar fashion, the brain stem—which, during REM sleep, delivers signs to soothe the muscles that are fundamental for body posture and limb movements so that we don't move around and act crazy while we dream—is also strongly impacted while a being works out. Physical exercise has been shown to induce various molecular and neuronal adaptations in the brain stem, which allows us to assume that the efforts made while strongly active can only aid the bottom portion of our brain as it runs during rest.

Other highly functioning areas in the brain during sleep include the hypothalamus, the thalamus, the pineal gland, and the basal forebrain, which are all affected, in one way or another, amidst a bouncy workout. While there is still a lot to learn about the true inner workings of sleep, and the basis of how and why dreams are cultivated, it is safe to surmise that positively strengthening the performance of regions in the brain while we exercise will naturally help those same sectors that have various responsibilities while we slumber.

Quite undeniably, if, on average, you routinely do not get the proper amount of rest, your mind and body will suffer drastically, which directly damages your ability to consistently succeed as a lively being. Drowsiness is detrimental to a soul who strives to shine, but beyond just feeling sleepy after a poor night's sleep, a shortage of solid shuteye has been proven to negatively affect one's memory, concentration, creativity, problem-solving skills, mood, balance, weight, immune system, and blood pressure, among other things. Inversely, a strong cycle of sleep has the ability to shift all the mentioned factors to the positive side of the spectrum, as it can enhance your attention, boost your immune system, improve your memory, and help with mood regulation. The more control we have over these factors, the more likely it is that we will increase our longevity and the overall time on Earth in which we are able to operate at our apex. Plus, from a physical standpoint, the better you are able to sleep, the easier it becomes for your muscles to effectively recover and grow. When you are inactive, your muscles discharge protein-building amino acids into your bloodstream at an enhanced rate, allowing them to ably amplify in size and strength. If you don't allow your body and mind to effectively recharge, you can't expect either of them to perform at a robust rate while you're actively operating in pursuit of your ambitions.

Now, I absolutely understand that getting an adequate amount of sleep sounds obvious to most, but, again, the population of preeminent people in our purview do the little things better than the average, and getting the right supply of rest is one of them. Putting the value of it into perspective, I want to share a study from the AAA Foundation for Traffic Safety. In the experiment, a group of researchers pulled sample data of police-reported crashes that took place between July 2005 and December 2007, and analyzed the connection between acute sleep deprivation and the odds that a drowsy, crash-involved driver had been at fault in a mix-up in which they were involved. Those supervising the study measured the number of hours that both the at-fault driver, and the faultless operator in an analyzed pileup, had slept in the past twenty-four hours, and took a total of 4,571 more-severe-than-average crashes into consideration for the test. "More severe than average" meant that all 4,571 shake-ups involved at least one car having to get towed due to damage and required support from emergency medical services (EMS). According to the results, those who had slept less than five hours in the past day were four times more likely to get into a crash than those who had slept at least eight hours. Even the individuals who reported getting seven hours of rest were twice as likely to be at fault in a smash-up as drivers who got eight or more hours.

This study is great because, not only was it the first to measure the connection between specific amounts of recent rest and the risk of causing an accident in a representative quantity of crashes amongst the general driving population, but it also helped illustrate, in numeric fashion, how lack of sleep can directly correlate to creating negative results for a being who is actively functioning. There has been a plethora of sponsored studies where researchers analyzed sleep and its relationship to athletic performance, or to test scores in the classroom, but the data within those areas could easily be skewed. If you're someone who has put in thousands of hours on the tennis court, meticulously molding your game, then operating on less or more sleep than usual might not matter as much because the objective of the sport is something you are incredibly familiar with and, most likely, skilled in. Plus, there are countless external factors that come into play when judging athletic conduct. The same thing goes for an exam in school. If a student has a strong understanding of the substance, then, as long as they are alert enough, they will presumably perform.

Analyzing car-wreck data in affiliation with sleep is arguably the strongest, most proper measurement to judge how amount of rest relates to performance because, inherently, no one, and I mean not one single soul, wants to be involved in an accident. For obvious reasons, the pressure to properly perform in any given trip is incomparable to practically all other fields that could be used to judge length of sleep as it's correlated to rate of success.

The purpose of alluding to the automobile accident data is not to alarm you, or make you believe that you must get a minimum of eight hours of sleep before even thinking about getting behind the wheel. It's simply referenced to exemplify how an inadequate amount of rest has the potential to lead to poor results in our reality. There are countless cases in this world that a lot of us have either experienced, personally seen, or heard about, where an individual emphatically succeeds in a specific endeavor with little to no rest. As we know, if you are able to align with the four, steadily harped-on rules for attainment, then anything is achievable. However, this book is built around taking the most effective actions possible, and, from a probability standpoint, in order to put yourself in the strongest position for realization in any effort, you must do your best to ensure that your inner battery is as close to 100 percent as humanly possible ahead of any significant undertaking.

So, is there a golden formula for dynamic rejuvenation that, if followed to a T, will galvanize our souls and max out our mental and physical attributes so that we can precisely prepare for a meaningful moment? Not exactly, but there are a handful of mechanisms that have been scientifically declared as efficacious options. Of course, there is a wave of epidemiological evidence that suggests, as an adult, getting seven to eight hours of sleep per night is most advantageous. Getting less than seven hours of rest on a consistent basis has been shown to lead to the previously referenced negative consequences that spawn when one is unable to get a suitable chunk of rest, and oversleeping on a regular cadence, while not as conclusive as the data from analyzing beings who get little to no rest, has been linked to both higher BMI and depression. If you're getting the advocated amount, that means you're already dedicating one-third of your existence to sleep, so don't get in a habit of excessive snoozing or you might take precious time away from your ambitions. Just for perspective purposes, let's say, as a functioning adult, you had a string of three years in which you averaged nine hours of sleep per night. If that was the case, then you have to live with the fact that you tossed 1,095 hours of your existence down the drain just to rest beyond the ideal recommendations. 1,095 hours that could have been used developing a skill, honing your craft, or creating timeless moments with friends and loved ones.

Outside of evaluating the optimal extent of inactivity that a being should strive for on a standard night, let's take a look at some alternative sleeping methods that have been practiced amongst those who aimed to religiously interact with reality at their mental and physical apex.

First up to bat, the timely stationed twenty-minute nap. Legend has it that both Leonardo da Vinci and Nikola Tesla faithfully followed a unique resting technique known as the Uberman cycle, which is a sleeping schedule consisting of six twenty-minute naps, evenly dispersed across a twenty-four-hour period. It has often been reported that da Vinci, while painting the eminent *Mona Lisa*, operated on this unorthodox method, as the Italian polymath, every four hours, would take a break from designing his iconic oil painting—featuring a seated, subtly smiling woman placed against an abstract landscape made up of valleys, mountains, hills, a river, and a bridge—and rest for twenty minutes before getting back to creating. If you do the quick math in your head, then you'll realize that da Vinci, if the tale is true, was inactive for only two hours per day, which, technically speaking, provided him with an additional six hours of productivity when in comparison to someone who sleeps the standard eight hours per day. Add this up over a protracted strand of years, and, if recurrently honored, which Tesla supposedly did throughout the majority of his existence, you'll hypothetically gain upwards of twenty years of active time to pursue your passions. However, if you're thinking about adopting this somewhat startling snoozing process in hopes of mimicking the production levels of da Vinci and Tesla, modern science strongly advises against it. Essentially all the research centered around the subject of polyphasic sleep raises extreme concerns, and is not recommended from a health, safety, or performance perspective.

For the best all-around results, subject-matter experts suggest sticking to a formal sleep pattern that allows you to get around eight hours of sleep, every twenty-four hours. Yet, along with resting through the night, another notable option for those jockeying to enhance their inherent mood and personal output is the daytime nap. Past studies designed around midday naps suggest that taking brief snoozes can positively impact one's alertness, cognitive function, self-confidence levels, and, from an overarching view, their ability to productively perform in an upcoming task that requires a mix of both physical and mental energy. World-class athletes, like Michael Jordan, LeBron James, Muhammad Ali, and Roger Federer, have been known to set aside time and briefly rest ahead of their respected events. For the best results, the National Sleep Foundation recommends taking a nap ranging between twenty and thirty minutes on any day that includes athletic competition.

Ultimately, when it comes to mapping out your sleep habits, aim for the eight hours, mix in a crisp nap where you can, but most importantly, find a way to systematically interact with the world at as close to 100 percent as possible. While we certainly cannot confidently declare that getting a minimal amount of sleep before an important action will directly lead to poor results, there is enough data out there that supports the benefits of getting the endorsed measure of rest. By partaking in an activity with feelings of fatigue, you are willingly transmitting only a portion of your potential energy. That statement alone should encourage all beings to fixedly focus on their sleeping routine.

This slice of the story was rather extensive because the quality of your inactive sessions directly correlates with the caliber of your active actions. If one-third of your existence is made up of an activity that has an immense influence on both your production levels and visible reality, then you must make sure you are constantly concentrated on that very act.

As has been highlighted, daily exercise will emphatically encourage both the body and mind to seek out rest, which, in turn, positively influences one's ability to effortlessly fall asleep, and helps them maintain an unshakeable run of inactivity throughout their dormant session. By elevating the inner workings that are in motion in the midst of a resting session, physically training is one of the strongest actions one can take on a consistent basis to establish a solid sleeping praxis. The better we sleep, the easier it is for our body to recharge and ultimately ripen, especially as it pertains to our muscles and mind. The more we feel at full strength, the more likely it is that we will succeed in any endeavor that calls for an orderly usage of our stamina.

Beyond just thinking about sleep as a means to revive the body, don't forget to aim your attention on the thoughts you have before dozing off. Historically, people just think about resting as an effective way to get their energy back and renovate their fibers, but in reality, there is so much more going on while our consciousness is suspended than we can ever imagine. While it sounds mystical, the referenced material at the top of the chapter strongly displayed how, when we focus on a problem or concept before knocking out, a solution for whatever it was that we were concentrated on gets sent to the brain in a magical manner. While the timing of when one awakes appears to correlate with the clarity of the thought, just knowing that a stretch of sleep has the power to help an individual uncover answers is wildly thrilling.

Before judging the validity of this claim, ponder over the pronounced powers that propagate from a mighty meditation practice. Introspection exercises are effective because the being is deliberately choosing to solely focus on their breathing, emotional scale, a personal mantra, a particular concept, or some blend of any of the four listed options. No matter the specifics, self-examination techniques work because, by erasing all things external for a brief moment, a conscious individual is able to enhance their clarity on whatever it is that they are focusing on, which allows them to drive forward with the mindset that will lead them to a solution. This is also the case when we lie down to rest. Your thoughts don't just go away when you fall asleep. They are still metaphorically floating around in your mind, except now, they are imagined with intense luminosity because of the substantial clean-up that is simultaneously occurring in your brain. As the brain tidies up and freshens its sectors, your mind is able to analyze your recent ideas with profound precision. This is why the individuals in the recalled experiments, and the aforementioned music artists, were effortlessly able to come to solutions on concepts that, immediately prior, had been giving them trouble.

So dream big, visualize with a clear intent, and ensure that your thoughts and emotions are in a positive place before dozing off. As the fortuitous conscious being, you are the one in charge of properly programming your brain. If you go to bed ruminating over an idea with a negative emotion attached to it, then you are voluntarily setting yourself up for future failure because, as your body goes to rest and the brain begins its purification process, the poor thought becomes magnified. Anytime an idea is amplified, whether good or bad, the brain formulates a path to creation.

Understanding this, it becomes ever-so-crucial that you go to bed with uplifting images symbolically sailing the seas of your psyche.

When it comes to tying your shoe, quite clearly, because of your assumed experience in the act, your level of vitality most likely will not alter the outcome, but, as your aims in life become more complex, the status of your present energy increases in importance as it relates to actualizing the result. Again, from a pure probability perspective, in order to put yourself in the strongest position for success in any endeavor that calls for physical or mental strength, you must do your best to ensure that you're at full capacity before putting energy into the action.

The same premise applies to the rules for achievement. Our quality of sleep primarily impacts the latter two regulations. Each time we take action toward our ambitions, our level of alertness has the power to strongly influence the outcome. The more energy spent in your desired space at full stamina, the less time, hypothetically, it will take to reach your fitting destination, as it's easiest to observe the potential alterations that you need to make when your body and mind are able to experience reality with acute clarity.

Since lack of sleep is capable of crippling both our moods and strength, one's self-confidence status can easily take a hit if an individual chooses to perform in a particular act with lackluster energy. Contrarily, getting an adequate amount of shuteye will undoubtedly heighten one's overall spirit and self-belief system, allowing them to enter any arena with the proper mindset for victory.

In a general sense, though not directly in cahoots with personal achievement, the better you sleep, the better you'll feel. Knowing the potency that sleep possesses in regard to shifting your reality and resetting your body, it is much more important than it's typically credited for. So don't overlook its immense value, and take the proper actions, like physically exercising in any fashion, to improve the process of falling asleep, and enhance the overall caliber of your resting session.

The last remark before climbing to the coming chapter is something to give thought to on a daily basis. Barring any present physical or mental injury, no matter how much energy you expend during your waking hours, your body and mind completely reset to full strength following a stable run of rest. Since all we have is the present moment, any amount of exertion that was not intently utilized yesterday is gone forever, and it can be properly viewed as wasted. Comprehending that everyone has an allegorical hourglass that topologically tracks their time in the flesh, in order to pull the most out of yourself in a confined amount of time, you must aim to discharge close to, if not all, of your stamina on as many of your active days as humanly possible.

Chapter 8

RATHER UNIQUE

A conventional characteristic that coincides with the cream-of-the-crop characters in this atmosphere is "strong ability to stand out amongst their field of competition." In other words, to be great, you must strive to be unparalleled by the people to the left and right of you. Since this project is all about living a healthy, cheerful, and luxurious life, I would like to spend some brief time discussing the benefits of being a one-of-a-kind individual and touch on how expressing originality directly leads to glory.

One's level of uniqueness as it pertains to success can be best envisioned in a theoretical field of nutritious apples. For this imagined scenery filled with nutrient-dense, round fruit, let's say that in one specific area, there is a blossoming tree bearing twelve equally sized apples that are freely growing and scattered evenly throughout the woody perennial plant. By chance, eleven of them are colored red, while the last of the set, for whatever odd reason, possesses a green pigment.

Let's pretend that you spawned into this symbolic scene and decided to head over to the referenced area. As you got closer to the tree, you began to observe it, and, after your brain quickly analyzed the pattern of red apples—as humans have a strong tendency to seek out specific arrangements for decision-making and educational purposes—you immediately concentrate all of your attention on the singular, grass-toned fruit. Since it's unlike the rest, and does not oblige to the sequence in the tree, your point of focus is zoomed in on the green one. After earnestly eyeing the healthy plant, you decide to make your way over to another sprouting seedling. By chance, this tree also has twelve apples, uniformly spread around its branches. However, as you start to closely evaluate it, you find that, unlike the previous piece of nature, all dozen of these apples are red. After spotting the orderliness, your focal point swiftly shifts to one specific, cardinal-colored pome fruit, located around the middle of the tree. This one, in particular, caught your attention because it is significantly bigger than its counterparts. In a similar sense, it's like the previously mentioned green apple, as it's comparable at its core to its peers, but possesses a strikingly different trait. Even though they are all the same product, the distinct size caused your brain to precisely fixate your attention on the largest one.

Following your evaluation, you head on over to a third tree. This one, by sheer coincidence, also includes a tally of twelve apples. Like the original tree, it has eleven red apples, and one green. As you promptly scan the tree, identifying the design that is predominately made up of red apples, you immediately become fascinated with the spinach-stained outlier. As you study it, you notice that, on top of its distinct color, the verdant-glowing apple is also significantly larger than its connected counterparts. Again, all the same product at heart, but the glaring uniqueness of the green one tugs the bulk of your attention toward it.

After appreciating the beauty of nature for a little bit longer, you were magically expunged from the field and returned to your previous location. Now, you're probably wondering what these allegorical apples have to do with this project and how this figure of speech relates to both fitness and personal attainment. You see, in life, in order to staunchly stand out amongst your contemporaries, you must aim to be the strongest, most potent apple within a group of matching fruit; a diverse, uniquely tinted, green apple surrounded by a spread of red; or a dynamic mixture of the two, meaning you are a supreme, one-of-a-kind green apple that is more tenacious, and rarer, than all of the red apples that you are surrounded by. If confused, here is a clear explanation of this metaphor:

In a field of rose-shaded apples, which is symbolic for your desired discipline, to be "extraordinary," you must aspire to be:

- **The biggest, most influential red apple:** Significantly more skilled than your peers.
- **A green apple:** Incredibly unique and creative, making you incomparable to your counterparts.
- **A durable, rarefied green apple:** A combination of the first two. Freakishly talented, while possessing strong

traits of originality, which makes you the preeminent, unrivaled being betwixt the competition.

Just as the human mind is naturally attracted to uniqueness, the universe, as a collective, is faithfully drawn to those who, in respect to their craft, are mightier, and, because of their harnessed, authentic talent, matchless to their associates. For this section, I will be solely focusing on standing out as a green apple, while the last chapter will highlight what it takes to be the most impactful red apple. To dwell as the impeccable combination of the two, simply organize your lifestyle around the included messages in the pair of segments.

To be the unique, green apple, we must first understand what it means to be regarded as "rare." Those who are considered "out of the ordinary" in a specific area of expertise, or even a social setting, typically possess an innovative taste, prolific mindset, and a strong drive to express themselves in a creative manner. Expressing your creative side is a precursor to transforming from a red apple to a green one. Whether it's standing out in a social circle, an artistic area, or in a business sense, those who attract attention and real recognition, aside from working hard and taking the necessary actions for success in their present pursuit, are the ones who emit their creative characteristics in whatever they are putting stamina toward. To not be creative is to remain a red apple, which is a metaphorical way of saying that, if you don't offer your ingenious energy to the world and all those around you, then you accept operating as a shell of yourself, and are completely fine with grouping up with a mass of people who are also opting to neglect their original elements. Since no two human beings are exactly alike, each and every one of us has something unique to gift the world; however, a large chunk of the population, for whatever reason, refuses to open their internal present.

Within our consciousness, we all have a creative side that, when tapped into, positively impacts our life in its entirety. Along with using your creativity to solve problems, expressing your inner ingenious character will promote feelings of happiness, enhance your self-esteem, aid in effective networking, fuel your drive to create, open up your eyes to potential opportunities, and ultimately, put you in a favorable position to become an innovative individual. Those who innovate are simply the ones who think outside of the box and create products or services that are considered "revolutionary" in comparison to the present option in the specific space, which is all just a fancy way of saying that innovative people exude their creative elements to further steer society in the right direction. Radiating your creative energy correlates with feelings of joy because you are literally grasping original matter from within and positively projecting it into reality. By pulling out whatever is in your heart, you'll naturally sense a wave of elation, which will inspire you to always keep going. Since the act of creating calls for materializing an intangible thought into a perceptible product or service, the road to realization is especially thrilling, as the invisible becomes visible in a magical manner.

As we've come to find out, consistently exercising will naturally boost your drive and point your state of mind in the right direction, but can it aid with cultivating creativity so that we are able to productively stick out amongst the herd? Of course.

In a 2014 study conducted by a group of researchers at Stanford University, 176 adults, the majority being college students, took part in a handful of exercises with the goal of the investigation being to further understand the possible connection between physical activity and creative thinking. To accurately analyze the potential findings, the participants were issued questions that called for creative analysis and were evaluated on said inquiries after a period of sitting, as well as following a leisurely walk.

To effectively measure ingenuity, the questions were based on divergent thinking. For those unfamiliar, divergent thinking is the process of producing multiple, unique explanations of a pending issue, or a general inquiry that one is aiming to solve. For example, a divergent thinking problem could be having to shout out, in a fixed amount of time, as many different ways one could effectively utilize a particular object as one could think of. If the object was newspaper, a list of appropriate answers could be to: serve as reading material, a book cover, window cleaning tool, or gift wrap.

Anyway, in one of the experiments, the participants were first tested while sitting down inside and then again while walking on a treadmill. The results showed that their creative output in the designated divergent thinking-centered assignment increased by an average of 60 percent amidst the light cardio session. The sheer act of moderately exercising appears to inject our brain with a healthy splash of creative juice that otherwise would not have been flushed into our mind, had we remained stagnant. Upon further analysis, the group of researchers also found that, even for a stretch of time after the walking drill, the individuals in the test kept their creative boost, which showed that you don't have to be simultaneously exercising and problem-solving to reap the creative jolt.

This of course makes complete sense, because when you do physically train, even if it's just a light stroll, you are naturally igniting sectors in your brain that, under immobile conditions, wouldn't have been stimulated. Yet this study in particular is epochal because it flagrantly illustrated how physically exercising sparked creative thoughts in active beings who, just prior to the movement, were unable to efficiently express the clever concepts buried in their brain. We already knew that working out boosts one's ability to effectively learn and retain information and reduces stress to promote mental clarity, but now knowing that it aids with unlocking our innovative ideas is incredibly intriguing.

As someone who is truly fascinated by analyzing successful
people with the hopes of mirroring their beneficial habits, when
I stumbled across this study, I began to wonder if notable figures
in this sphere had consciously, or unconsciously, incorporated
some form of physical exercise into their lifestyle amidst a
creative undertaking. Interestingly enough, it turns out that some
of the more well-known visionaries in this world have in fact
taken advantage of the creative clarity that emanates through
the encephalon as a result of physical movement. Steve Jobs
was known for conducting "walking meetings" where he and
his employees, colleagues, or potential partners would saunter
around Apple's neighborhood in Cupertino, California, and
vividly discuss their ideas for innovation. Ernest Hemingway, the
renowned American novelist who penned *The Old Man and the
Sea*, which won the Pulitzer Prize for Fiction in 1953, like Jobs,
took full advantage of the creative spark that blossoms into the
conscious mind through exercise, as the acclaimed author was an
avid hiker.

In the music space, amidst recording his fifth studio album, *My
Beautiful Dark Twisted Fantasy*, which won Best Rap Album
at the 2012 Grammy Awards, Kanye West and his artistic
collaborators would routinely set aside some time each day to
lift weights and play basketball together before heading over to
the studio to work on the symphonic adventure that wound up
manifesting as a musical masterpiece. While putting together
melodic gems, Ludwig van Beethoven, German composer, would

often take spirited walks after he ate lunch. Along these spunky strolls, he would carry a pencil and a few sheets of paper with him to properly document any musical thoughts that happened to brightly burst into his conscious mind as he opened up his soul to the sensational surroundings of the great outdoors, and soaked up the ever-so-potent vitamin D from the sunlight.

Over in the movie world, in a similar light, Quentin Tarantino, the illustrious filmmaker who has written and directed a multitude of memorable motion pictures, most recently *Once Upon a Time in Hollywood*, *The Hateful Eight*, and *Django Unchained*, when asked about his creative process in a 2021 interview on *The Joe Rogan Experience*, mentioned that, after voraciously writing for a stretch of hours in the daytime, he likes to "hop in his pool and just kind of float around in the warm water and think about everything I've just written." According to the moviemaker himself, as he swims, ingenious ideas begin to profoundly pop into his head, which allows him to, upon exiting the pool, scribble down some key notes to carry momentum into the next scripting session.

Apprehending this, if you're yearning to stick out in a creativity-centered craft, you must concentrate on consistently staying active while shaping your creation. Even though the connection between unique thinking and physical exercise is not as popularized as some of the other perks that come along with working out, it is quite clear that individuals, when attempting to express their creative ideas, are at a significant advantage when they set aside time to put their body in motion, in comparison to those who pursue artistic endeavors while living a sedentary life. Creatives use art to broadcast, in remarkable fashion, intricate imaginative abstractions in a sensible manner, and the only way to align with this quest is through strong problem-solving ability, tip-top observational capacity, mighty recollection strength, elite idea-formation, and supreme diverse-thinking skills, which are all attributes that are amplified through physical fitness.

Even if you don't aspire to operate in an artistically based setting, enhancing your ability to think creatively will naturally place you in a prime position to effectively distinguish your character from the masses, which is something all of us should steadily strive for. At our core, whether we verbally admit it or not, we all want to be recognized and deeply appreciated for the way we go about our business in this three-dimensional space, and the easiest way to align with that mission is by keenly concentrating on how we can express ourselves in the most original and compelling way possible. If you routinely spend your days moving and thinking in a mundane manner, your allegorical apple, symbolic of you as a person, will remain an ordinary red pigment, while those who focus on rescuing their creative characteristics from the depths of their psyche will, figuratively, get greener, and literally, stick out like the sour sensation that one sharply senses after consuming a grass-shaded lime.

Running with this metaphor, quickly think about your friends, loved ones, and all the individuals that you admire in this atmosphere. The feeling of affinity that you have toward them stems from your ability to see their unique characteristics. Had there been nothing on the surface that separates their personality and output from the common person, you wouldn't sense the same level of appreciation for them, just as your eyes do not value a red apple mixed in with other cardinal-colored apples.

Keep in mind that, no matter the severity of the physical drill, as long as you're mobile in some form or fashion, the injection of ingenuity will always be effectively infused. A good chunk of the exercise examples above, along with the workout in the scientific study, lean heavily toward the lighter side in reference to level of wear and tear on the body, which tells us that, as long as we are moving, we will inherently secure the benefits. That right there is the most important point that I'm trying to get across in this specific section and, truthfully, the project in its entirety. The brain that dwells in a static being is not the same vast engine that resides, and rapidly runs, in a physically active individual. When you're stagnant, blood flows into your brain at a gradual speed, which is a major disservice to your brain cells, as these units of intellectual power rely heavily on the oxygen and nutrients within the blood in order to effectively perform at a high rate. Prior research has shown that when your blood flows at a snail-like pace, as a result of remaining in a static position, it is quite common for your thinking prowess to be briefly blurred.

In addition, scientists have also discovered that spending long periods in a stationary position will lead to thinning of the brain's medial temporal lobe, a region within the cerebral cortex that is vital to memory development. So when we read about these studies that involve individuals improving their ability to think creatively either while, or shortly after, exercising, the drastic change in results should come as no surprise, because these beings were literally operating with a completely different power source than when they were tested while sitting. One is a clouded, inefficient instrument, while the other is a mighty motor that is clicking on all cylinders. With that said, if you live a primarily parked lifestyle, you must accept that fact that your brain will never function at its apex, which of course means you will never tap into the boundless potential that is naturally ingrained in each one of us.

As our goal posts in life extend farther and farther, it is ever-so-important that we have full command over what we can control. This calls for ensuring that our bodies and minds are regularly placed in the strongest position possible ahead of any meaningful life event. By comprehending the fact that your brain will not think as clearly, or cleverly, when your body is habitually, or presently, in an idle state, you must continually focus on being as active as humanly possible if you wish to consume the immeasurable brilliance that dwells within the heart of your intelligence.

The purpose of perpetually penning these motivational tidbits throughout the project is not to push you in a certain direction, or to come across as a preacher. This story is simply a mix of concrete science, evidence/research-based studies, social examples, and a small dose of philosophy to further drive home the outlined information. According to the numbers, present-day people are spending more time in sedentary positions than ever before, and this trend doesn't appear to be slowing down anytime soon. After pulling data (on nearly 52,000 people from 2001 to 2016) provided by the National Health and Nutrition Examination Survey (NHANES), Yin Cao, an assistant professor in public health sciences at the Washington University School of Medicine, and a group of additional colleagues found that, on average, teens and young adults in 2016 spent an hour more each day in a seated position than adolescents did in 2007. And it's not like the next generation is specifically setting aside time each day to partake in some type of seated meditation practice. 62 percent of the kids from 2016, ages five to eleven, were recorded spending at least two hours a day sitting in front of the TV or perched in front of a computer, watching videos online. From a purely structural standpoint, since regular exercise has the wondrous ability to increase the size of specific regions in the brain correlated with learning, decision-making, and other vital human processes, one could certainly presume that constant sitting is especially bad for children, as the brain grows at an astonishing rate during our early years.

Beyond kids, the statistics also revealed that 50 percent of adults
in 2016, outside of work or school, spent at least one hour per day
of their leisure time sitting in front of the computer screen, which
was a staggering increase in comparison to the grownups in 2003,
a year in which only 29 percent of adults spent sixty or more
minutes on a computer in their free time.

Now, quite obviously, time spent sitting can of course be used for
personal development and mood-enhancing purposes, but with
the incredible popularity surge of video games, endlessly growing
amount of non-beneficial content getting published by the
second, progressively worse diets that lead to lazy habits, and the
sheer, borderline-unhealthy, obsession with continually staying
connected to society by way of an electronic device, increasing
our hours spent in a sedentary position, as we've come to find out,
directly harms our ability to think critically and creatively. When
you think about the most iconic works of art in human history,
the creations that come to mind—like *The School of Athens* by
Raphael, *The Thinker* by Rodin, the aforementioned *Mona Lisa*
by Leonardo da Vinci, Michelangelo's work on the ceiling of the
Sistine Chapel, Pablo Picasso's *Guernica*, and Vincent van Gogh's
The Starry Night—were all created in eras with no internet, and
in times when the average human being was forced to remain on
their feet much more often than present-day folks.

So, if you ever read about incredibly ingenious periods in human
history, like the Old Kingdom of Egypt (2700–2200 BCE), ancient

Greece (500–336 BCE), ancient Rome (eighth century BCE to late fourth century CE), the Italian Renaissance (fourteenth to seventeenth century CE), Louis XIV's reign in France (1638–1715), or the Age of Enlightenment in Western Europe and beyond (1685–1815), always keep in the back of your mind that during these tidal waves of artistic innovation, people were habitually on their toes, effortlessly allowing the creative juices to flood their consciousness.

With all this being said, I don't necessarily believe that society is doomed, or that we are in serious trouble, from an innovation standpoint, if we continue this trend of spending less and less time on our feet. In the last fifty years alone, we have seen the invention, and incredible evolution, of the cellphone, the digital camera, Automated Teller Machines, electric cars, photovoltaic solar energy, bar codes and scanners, and online shopping, to name a few. Not to mention the unprecedented strides in the medical world.

Additionally, as you're reading this, there has never been a better time in human history to efficiently consume beneficial information, connect with potent people, and ultimately get your vision out to the masses. Plus, the sheer amount of continuously growing raw data allows us to push on in the information age. Because of this, there will always be outliers in the culture who change the world. Yet, one could very well argue that, based on what we know about the issues that come with living a sedentary lifestyle, we humans, as a collective, could be wildly more effective and creative if we sat less and moved more.

～

Along with driving the development of deeper social connections, aiding in your pursuit to conceive timeless art, elevating your personal brand, boosting your internal morale, increasing your drive, putting you in a position to make a profound impact in a team environment, or naturally improving your ability to thrive in a behavior-based setting, expressing your creative side, at its crux, helps you find you. The more energy you expend trying to fit in a box with the rest of society, the less time you will spend as the original character that you were wondrously designed to be, which is why it is vital to make a concerted effort to find areas that you're fond of and symbolically spray them with your exclusive astuteness.

Did you know that, with an average shoe, one with six pairs of eyelets, there are nearly two trillion sequences that one could follow to effectively feed the laces through the twelve eyelets? Two trillion. When it comes to tying them, there are a variety of ways to accomplish this feat as well. All this to say, there are an immeasurable number of routes that one could take in life, yet the majority of people carelessly walk the path most taken, which symbolically results in bland piles of red apples getting sadly spread all across the world.

Simply put, if you do not express your unparalleled ideas and creative ingenuity, you are hurting both yourself and society. Our inherent hourglass that measures our time in the flesh never stops, so focus, in real time, on creating, because those who express themselves, whether it be physically in a performance act, uniquely in an artistic arena, or distinctively in a business setting, live on forever as unprecedented green apples amongst a group of reds.

Swooping in our recipe for achievement, one's level of creativity plays a role in each of the four ingredients. Depending on the actual objective, the resources needed to fulfill specific feats can easily vary. Creative people in this reality find ways to either use their supplies in unique fashion, or include additional means to further enhance their ability to stand out. Strong creative-thinking skills lead to an augmentation in one's capacity to think outside of the box, which matters greatly in areas where competition is steep, and suitable spots are limited. When it comes to clearly understanding the outcome of a certain mission, an ingenious individual will most likely strive to achieve the desired aim in the most original way possible.

The actions taken by visionaries, while at times similar to those in their space, are, in the long run, recognizably distinctive from the plurality of people in their discipline. Incredibly ingenious individuals plot out their daily moves and are supremely focused on constantly putting energy toward their craft which, in due time, leads to an exclusive personification of their prolific thoughts. As a constant reminder, the more active you are amidst your specific undertaking, the more valuable your actions become, especially if your endeavor is creativity-centered. It is quite clear that when you are motionless, not only do your muscles rest, but so too does your brain, which directly inhibits your ability to maximize your intelligence in the moment. It is practically impossible to reach great heights using just a slice of the infinite potential that is marvelously planted within your cranium, so, for the best results, stay on your toes, in real time, during creation. Even if you've already exercised for the day, if you're ever struggling to extract your internal wisdom in times where you are searching for answers, focus on the current questions, and, simultaneously, get moving.

Finally, the more authentic matter you express outward, the higher your level of self-confidence will be, as creatively communicating your inner character translates to you effectively existing as yourself, which naturally elevates your level of assurance in your ability to achieve whatever it is that you decide to put energy toward.

On the whole, next time you're physically active, do yourself a favor, and crack a nice smile. Not just because you're enhancing your physical being, boosting your intellect, uplifting your spirit, elevating your ability to dwell in the present, putting yourself in a strong position for a great night's sleep, improving your breathing habits, and promoting your desire to set goals, but because you're literally unlocking your creative excellence, allowing you to smoothly separate yourself from the pack, and swimmingly attract authentic adoration from all those around.

Chapter 9

KEEP SHOWING UP

To be the mightiest, most dynamic red apple amongst your counterparts, you must outwork everyone in your chosen field. In any performance-based pursuit, or really any especial area in which your level of efficiency matters greatly when it comes to continually creating the desired results, the more work you put in, the easier it is to effectively produce. For competitive settings that call for extreme proficiency in behavior, the harder one works in comparison to the field, the more fear they are able to inject into the psyche of the opposition, giving them an increased advantage in the heart of a clash.

Symbolically visualizing yourself as an apple, each time you put energy toward your goals, the larger, and more tasteful your emblematical, edible form becomes, allowing you to break from the band and considerably boost your odds for achievement. Aside from death and taxes, an additional guarantee in life that should be routinely grouped with the aforementioned pair is the fact that, each time you put stamina toward something, your level of understanding in that act increases. While the specifics of the action carry immense weight in regard to how much you will actually improve within each effort, no matter what, every time you focus on an explicit interest, you will undoubtedly increase your level of awareness in that area, which naturally elevates your odds of achieving success in that space.

The power source within our cranium, conventionally known as the brain, is programmed to attentively absorb whatever we focus on, and expertly store all the incoming information in a way that allows us, as conscious beings, to utilize the knowledge in the most beneficial, emotionally pleasing manner possible. In other words, your brain is magnificently built for you to win.

This can be best explained and envisioned through some brief science. Years ago, neuroscientists used to believe that, once we moved on from our adolescent stage in life, our brain stopped developing. However, because of the research conducted in the last fifty-odd years, experts can now confidently state that the brain, at any point in life, has the ability to modify and alter its programming as part of a reaction to any sensed experience. In scientific terms, this understanding is known as "neuroplasticity." Without this inherent process, humans wouldn't be able to show any signs of intellectual advancement as they progress through life.

Neuroplastic modification materializes at the chemical, structural, and functional levels of the brain. When you start learning something new, you will see the chemical change, which positively impacts your short-term memory and short-term ability in the specific feat. As you put in more time on the act, gaining a better understanding of how to effectively generate the right results, your brain will undergo a structural shift, one where your neurons will revise their connections. This new arrangement influences your memory and understanding from a long-term perspective. Once a considerable amount of time and energy is put toward the action, there will be a functional change, which allows a being to become incredibly efficient and skilled in whatever it was that they opted to repeatedly focus on.

This tectonic transformation has been observed firsthand in a handful of studies, yet, most notably, in one led by Earl K. Miller, a neuroscience professor at the Massachusetts Institute of Technology. In the examination, Miller and his research team analyzed monkeys and provided them with a very basic drill involving two photos. If picture A was presented, the monkey was instructed to look to the left; if picture B, to the right. If the long-tailed primates performed the task correctly, meaning they glanced in the direction that was in accordance with the photo, they were gifted some ever-so-tasty juice as a way to signify success. Throughout the test, the group of researchers were tracking brain function of the tree-climbing participants.

Following the experiment, Miller was quoted as saying, "neurons in the prefrontal cortex and striatum, where the brain tracks success and failure, sharpened their tuning after success." With the enhancement that resulted from flourishing in the act, the researchers also found that the neurological tune-up remained for several seconds after, which allowed the monkeys to improve with each subsequent attempt, and ultimately succeed more efficiently. What's interesting about this examination is that, when the monkeys failed in their attempt to look the right way when the picture was presented, there was little to no change in brain activity, which tells us that the brain is essentially wired to stockpile only the information necessary for benefit, allowing us mammals to constantly advance each time we put energy toward a specific act or subject.

As alluded to earlier, physically exercising is arguably the strongest action that one could consistently take in order to gain an apparent appreciation of how success is molded into the brain. After every training session, an active being can physically feel their body getting stronger and healthier, while also sensing the emotional boost that spawns from an effortful workout. This process subconsciously tells our brain that putting in physical work generates positive results, allowing us to mentally label each workout as an accomplishment.

Staying on this train of thought, one of the more under-appreciated, yet beautiful, aspects of physically exercising is the fact that every tallied workout is truthfully an inherent victory. Even on days when you don't feel at your best, and know that you could have performed at a higher level, the mere act of functional training, beyond the results, equips you with so many physical and mental boosts that it's practically impossible not to classify every session as an innate win. For the majority of actions that we take on any given day, the outcome of the act strongly determines our level of satisfaction, whereas energy put toward fitness automatically creates positive feelings and a sense of achievement. As touched on earlier, when we exercise, we actively release endorphins, oxytocin, dopamine, and serotonin, which are all also naturally discharged whenever we happily succeed at something in our day-to-day life. This means that we can mirror the feeling of a personal, social, or career highlight just by participating in a fitness workout. That basis right there is much more important than it is typically given credit for, because the more success we sense, the more confident we become, which allows us to systematically move forward in life with unshakeable faith in whatever we do. Plus, the dopamine kick felt from thriving in an event is addictive, which, in this sense, is incredibly positive and naturally primes a being to chase the sensation on a consistent basis. So, scientifically speaking, regularly exercising, because of its direct connection to success, empowers a being to habitually feel, and dwell as, a prizewinning specimen.

This is so vital because, to consistently conquer our goals, we must steadily stand as almighty spirits. To accomplish this, we must first physically sense the strength within. If you do not feel like a blooming being, it becomes very difficult to confidently put energy into anything that requires physical and mental stamina. Once we feel victorious, all we have to do is put in the work to correctly wire our brain so that our being is naturally placed in a winning position in whatever we choose to do. Knowing what we know, if you were to exercise every single day, whether it be cardio, strength, flexibility, balance, or coordination-based, you would precisely exist as a champion on a constant cadence, which would accurately arm you with the mental and physical moxie to achieve whatever you desire.

Additionally, if you choose to customarily work out, no matter how you feel on any given day, over time, your deliberate decision will naturally shift to an automatic practice. In plain terms, this is known as "developing a habit." While overanalyzed, the science of forming strong habits is a lot simpler than society makes it out to be. To create positive patterns, all you have to do is repeat a beneficial behavior over and over in the same framework, and, without even having to think, the control of your action instinctively transfers from something that was consciously directed, to something that is subconsciously sparked by conditional or circumstantial signals. In the brain, the initial choice to partake in an action is aligned with the prefrontal cortex, the area in your brain responsible for decision-making, but, as you routinely put in the time and shift it to an innate habit, the behavior becomes symbolically cemented into your basal ganglia, the part of your brain that is correlated with pattern recognition. This is crucial to comprehend because the formation of a habit translates to an automated action, which means you don't have to think about doing it, giving your prefrontal cortex a rest. When this occurs, an active being is able to allot their mental energy toward external happenings despite presently operating in a specific effort, which essentially provides the individual with supplementary stamina. This is easiest to visualize when brushing your teeth or tying your shoes. In both acts, because they are daily habits that have been performed countless times, you don't have to put mental thought toward the objectives, allowing your brain to focus on other, more important, manifestations amidst the efforts.

Once working out becomes part of your daily routine, because of its magical ability to adequately arrange your physical and emotional levels, you'll naturally be inclined to breed other helpful habits into your day-to-day lifestyle, in hopes of stimulating the same sensations sensed from exercising. This is why individuals who constantly exercise are, on average, happier and healthier than those who are predominately inactive. Apart from the perceptible improvement in one's mood and strength, the construction of the productive habit, which is daily exercise, encourages energetic individuals to map out their remaining waking hours with similar practices that provide their soul with more positive feelings. Once additional salubrious tendencies are fixed into your regular schedule, it becomes incredibly easy to live a merry life, because an agenda filled with positive habits means you are spending more time in the moment, enjoying your actions, and little to no time using your prefrontal cortex to overthink about your existence and worry about making certain

decisions. A life comprised of strong, healthful habits enhance
one's dopamine, serotonin, oxytocin, and endorphin levels,
creating a happy soul who is scientifically seeded with the secret
sauce to subsist as a profoundly productive person.

While this may sound too good to be true, it's really just science,
and the fact of the matter is, most people don't take the time out
of their day to plan their waking hours in accordance with what
they love, and what will truly take them to the next level. If your
day is entirely made up of actions that provide you with joy, that
are also of benefit for your personal growth, as you continuously
participate in this pleasurable program, these events become
ingrained in your basal ganglia, and, inherently, your pattern of
choice becomes who you are.

In a sheer identical light, along with molding physical patterns
into the mind, conscious beings are also able to implant any
mental ideas that they would like woven into their belief system
for good. Whether the thought is based on your self-worth, or
what you believe to be possible for you to achieve in this life, if
you get in the habit of projecting positive notions about yourself,
your abilities, and the aims that you will bring to fruition,
these beneficial beliefs will naturally become rooted into your
psyche. All you have to do is put in the time to transmit these
thoughts, over and over, and, eventually, what was once a concept
ruminating in your prefrontal cortex is now a fixed fact securely
stashed in your individual mental outlook. So constantly tell

yourself exactly what your ideal being would say to themselves in a self-talk session and, in due time, you will be one with this warrior. As mentioned earlier, to become your optimal character, simply self-identify with that entity, emulate their actions, and, as time prolongs, you'll naturally morph into the desired prototype.

To make the quest to becoming the quintessential more enjoyable, construct an agenda that is filled with assignments that will, number one, help you on your journey to becoming the ideal, and, number two, be doable enough that you are able to regularly feel the sense of attainment as the mission is completed. As active beings, the more work we complete, the better we feel, and, thankfully, we have full control over what can be defined as "work." Being conscious means that we have the ability to mentally create a list of things to do, that, when realized, because we defined the effort as a direct undertaking, provide us with an emotional boost. Every time we check something off our to-do list, whether it be basic responsibilities like taking out the trash or going to the grocery store, or more laborious tasks like running two miles or writing a thousand words for a book project, no matter what, upon fulfilment, we are awarded an innate sense of satisfaction for merely completing an act that we had specifically set out to do. Knowing this, in real time, to uplift your existence, you should constantly create personal chores so that your brain is programmed to routinely generate sunny feelings that correspond with achievement.

Further examining the referenced study at the top of the chapter, one could confidently conclude that the test monkeys were more inclined to succeed in the act because of the tasty liquid that was supplied to them following a fitting bid. As humans, we know this to be accurate because, whenever we see or mentally project an award that awaits our success in a particular act, our brain acknowledges the desired prize and methodically discharges an enhanced amount of dopamine, further promoting our drive and motivation to get the job done. Beyond the labor that stands between you and an achievement, establishing an award to be obtained prior to the fulfilment of an objective can be utilized across all areas of your life, no matter the ensuing act. For example, one, borderline-ludicrous, habit that I have set in stone is, each morning, before I'm allowed to eat my breakfast, I have to do twenty-five ab-rollouts using my ab wheel. With the prize being a heavenly feast comprised of a flavorful, fruit-and-yogurt smoothie and a plate of freshly cooked egg whites sprucely braided with spinach, I inherently become more inspired to complete the physical exercise so that I'm able to promptly reap the savory reward. Additionally, because the action in the way of the award is fitness-based, I'm able to collect the natural kick of neurotransmitters so that, upon completion, the garnered serotonin and oxytocin allows me to enjoy the meal even more. Setting a reward to receive following the fulfilment of a mundane act is one thing, but when the effort involves physically exercising, you're able to innately appreciate it twice as much because of the additional release of the positive chemical substances, which, immediately, raises your mood, lowers your stress levels, and upgrades your executive function skills. So from a scientific perspective, if you're aiming to revel-in an upcoming occurrence to the fullest, whether it be a date with your significant other, hanging with friends, watching a movie, or something as simple as eating a nice meal, work out immediately prior to the affair so that you can inherently receive the mighty jolt of serotonin and oxytocin, giving your soul a boost in mood and overall adoration for your existence and all those around. If physically exercising precisely promotes your state of mind and overall capacity to love, why wouldn't you participate in a fitness drill right before putting energy toward something that you long to deeply appreciate? Just something to keep in mind if you're ever looking for ways to further enjoy specific events in your human experience.

So design your life around activities that boost your being, make sure to constantly put action toward everything that you wish to excel in, create personal prizes, and, always make fitness a top priority, because the act of physical movement is an extraordinary exercise that results in a soul-sensed victory every single time. Knowing that there's a natural action out there that guarantees a sense of success, and instantaneously puts you in a winning spirit, you must take full advantage of it, and the more you do so, the more natural it'll feel to dwell as a victorious individual. Once your body and mind are permanently placed in a triumphant zone, you can seamlessly exist as the ideal version of yourself by purely putting energy toward anything in life that you aspire to flourish in. The more successful you feel, the easier it is to progress in whatever area you're focused on, so keep showing up to exercise, and you'll never have to worry about the status of your physical and mental health getting in the way of your ambitions.

This final section comes packed with a repetitive emphasis on the importance of daily exercise, and a tone with a serious sense of urgency because the truth is, your body and mind will peak at some point or another. While there are certainly some outliers out there defying the odds in both departments, it is clear that one's athletic ability and cognitive strength will progressively increase, hit a climax, and gradually worsen in a number of areas as time prolongs. Comprehending this concrete fact, it is ever-so-imperative that you attentively maximize your inherent powers by ensuring all the energy you expend is in accordance with your personal goals, and the easiest way to remain in alignment with this aim is by regularly exercising to accumulate the native boosts, and dressing your day with potent practices that will propel you toward your dreams and aspirations. Those who truly grind, day in and day out, don't spend an iota of time thinking about what they could have done better with their past energy, while those who knowingly coast by with haphazard effort put themselves at serious risk to undergo years of regret once reality seeks in and their once-desired opportunity is only observable in the rearview mirror of a vehicle that is unable to go in reverse.

Above all the inspirational talk, what's essential to understand is that the more energy put toward a particular area, the more information your brain is able to effectively store for your benefit, which allows you to, over time, get progressively more and more comfortable with classifying yourself as "successful" in that specific space. You are truly just a manifestation of your daily habits, so sketch out a schedule solely comprised of efforts that your optimal self would partake in, and, most importantly, to ensure that you habitually interface with the world as a happy, healthy, strong, loving, driven, and successful soul, keep exercising.

When it comes to tying your shoe, the act, at this point in your existence, is rather effortless, solely because of the number of times you have tackled the task. Your brain has mastered the art of lacing up your kicks, and permanently stored the solution, allowing you to exist on autopilot amidst the operation. To improve in any area of life, reflect on your road to shoe-tying excellence, and mirror the path by continuing to show up.

In reference to the compound for continual consummation, this chapter concentrates candidly on rule number three, "Take consistent action to further improve your success rate when performing the act." With each subsequent stab, your brain gains an increasingly better understanding of the effort, allowing your soul to advance with ease in the specific undertaking. Remember, by way of magic, your encephalon is wondrously assembled for you to achieve all of your ambitions. All you have to do is live by the rules, and intently focus on putting energy toward your objectives until you cross the finish line.

Exercise plays a direct role in your level of consistency because the more you physically train—because of the discharge of dopamine—the stronger your drive will be to punctiliously pursue your desires. On top of jacking up your will to work, by routinely exercising—meaning you are constantly participating in an act that regularly results in an inevitable victory upon completion—you are communicating to your brain, over and over, that you're a successful soul, which truly sets the table for you to expertly attack whatever you choose to put on your plate.

Above all, when it comes to comprehending the worth of physical exercise when paired with your ability to accomplish your goals, take a second and imagine there was a magic pill that could marvelously place your being in the strongest position possible to smoothly succeed in manifesting all of your intentions. For this capsule of medicine to be continuously classified as "effective," it would have to be able to elevate your mental clarity, ramp up your will, heighten your focus, expand your ability to think creatively, boost your self-belief status, station your soul in a success-sensing state, raise your capacity to love, help you swimmingly shift into your unconscious element for striking energy rejuvenation, encourage you to aim for specific targets, and ultimately increase the odds for you to remain healthy enough to put stamina toward any effort. As it wonderfully turns out, this supernatural supplement already exists, and has been on the market for as long as we've been conscious. To take it, and reap all of the astounding benefits, all you have to do is recurrently exercise in any fashion. From there, once the dynamic tablet is symbolically consumed, focus on what makes you happy, continue to show up, and watch your dreams unfold in ways that you personally couldn't even imagine.

AFTERWORD

Physical exercise is arguably the most miraculous action that one could consciously put energy toward on a consistent basis because all of the noted advantages that hatch within your personage, as a result of sensibly pushing your being, systematically spawn upon fulfilment of the act. Not a single thought, or ounce of stamina, needs to go toward trying to acquire the referenced perks. All you have to do is show up, and do the work. Turn physical fitness into a habit, and the omnipotent benefits are yours for keeps.

As we rapidly approach the finish line, my hope at this point in the race is that, moving forward, you figuratively carry these transcendent elements with you for the next time you feel fatigued amidst a spirited workout. While withdrawing every last piece of strength from the depths of your soul to successfully complete the session, keep in mind why you're doing it. Exercising isn't just about enhancing your visible appearance and improving your physical skills. It's about morphing into your superhuman self by revving up the almighty motor in your head so that you're able to energetically storm toward your goals and aspirations with a power source that's packed with limitless potential.

Before closing up this treatise for good, a few words of wisdom that I've found to be quite beneficial while I saunter on my human odyssey. First and foremost, self-discipline is the most dynamic trait that one can develop when on the path to prominence.

Secondly, if you consistently put energy toward your present goals and whatever areas that make you happy, it becomes increasingly more difficult to live with regret as time prolongs. While aligning with this aim, try your best to live in the moment, and don't ever forget that your brain is designed for you to dominate.

Thirdly, while on your personal journey, focus heavily on the work. When your attention is solely on the details, you're able to avoid putting any negative light on the ideal result, which allows your brain to naturally flock toward the optimal objective, as it is wide-open and unharmed. Additionally, while hard to accurately explain, when you zero in on your efforts, your passage will become watered with magic-like happenings, allowing the actual materialization of a specific desire to be ten times better than you could have ever envisioned.

Last but not least, if you ever feel lost, or lose faith in your ability to create your perfect reality, take a deep breath, and look down at your shoes. Remember, if you can tie your shoes, you can do anything. If you own the appropriate resources, have a clear understanding of the ideal outcome, take consistent action to further improve your success rate when performing in the act, and, most importantly, carry an unshakeable belief in your ability, so much so that you're fully convinced you've already flourished in the feat, then the world is yours.

Peace and Love.

FUNCTIONAL TRAINING FOR THE MIND SOUNDTRACK

For Spotify and/or Apple Music users,

Please scan the appropriate QR code below to unlock the official soundtrack for *Functional Training for the Mind*. The selected songs for the playlist each represent a separate section within the story.

Beyond listening to the tabbed tunes for pure enjoyment purposes, or even as fuel to energetically propel you through a demanding workout, I hope that each time one of these melodies hits your ears, you'll be robustly reminded of the immeasurable strength you possess inside.

Apple Music

Spotify

ABOUT THE AUTHOR

Jeremy Bhandari (born June 19, 1996) is an American author who pens projects that are specifically cultivated to help the reader become the best version of themselves. Aside from writing, he focuses on spreading love and positivity. When it comes to this experience as a whole, Jeremy puts a heavy emphasis on the importance of fitness, eating right, and taking genuine interest in those around you.

Twitter: @ JeremyBhandari

Instagram: Jeremy__Bhandari

Website: realjeremy.com (Subscribe to Newsletter & Check for Merch!)

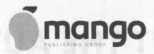

Mango Publishing, established in 2014, publishes an eclectic list of books by diverse authors—both new and established voices—on topics ranging from business, personal growth, women's empowerment, LGBTQ+ studies, health, and spirituality to history, popular culture, time management, decluttering, lifestyle, mental wellness, aging, and sustainable living. We were recently named 2019 *and* 2020's #1 fastest-growing independent publisher by *Publishers Weekly*. Our success is driven by our main goal, which is to publish high-quality books that will entertain readers as well as make a positive difference in their lives.

Our readers are our most important resource; we value your input, suggestions, and ideas. We'd love to hear from you—after all, we are publishing books for you!

Please stay in touch with us and follow us at:

Facebook: Mango Publishing
Twitter: @MangoPublishing
Instagram: @MangoPublishing
LinkedIn: Mango Publishing
Pinterest: Mango Publishing
Newsletter: mangopublishinggroup.com/newsletter

Join us on Mango's journey to reinvent publishing, one book at a time.